New Techniques in Tissue Surgery

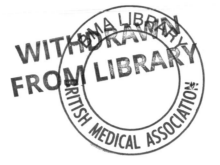

Maria Z. Siemionow (Ed)

Tissue Surgery

With 100 Figures

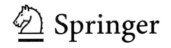
Springer

Maria Z. Siemionow, MD, PhD, DSc
Director of Plastic Surgery Research
Head, Microsurgery Training
Department of Plastic Surgery
The Cleveland Clinic Foundation
Cleveland OH
USA

British Library Cataloguing in Publication Data
A catalogue record for this book is available from the British Library

Library of Congress Control Number: 2005928176

ISBN-10: 1-85233-970-5   e-ISBN: 1-84628-128-8
ISBN-13: 978-1-85233-970-8

Printed on acid-free paper

Printed in the Singapore   (BS/KYO)

9 8 7 6 5 4 3 2 1

Springer Science+Business Media
springeronline.com

Preface

I was very enthusiastic when I was approached in November 2004 to edit a book on tissue surgery in the *New Techniques in Surgery* series. I was convinced that it would be great to have a book in a collection that so elegantly shows the progress in our understanding, handling, and approach to different types of tissues. The greatest challenge was to ensure that the title, *New Techniques,* was not misleading. My goal was to find creative contributors willing to share their novel techniques, while at the same time ensuring that the techniques were up-to-date at the time of publication. To achieve this goal, book production could not exceed one year and the contributors had to commit to share their most innovative approaches to tissue surgery while maintaining scheduled deadlines. This was a challenging task, but my collaborative efforts in the field over past decade enabled me to find creative and supportive surgeons who met those requirements. Finally, the presentation of new techniques in surgery had to be supported by the experience and reputation of the surgeons who introduced them.

The title of the book, *Tissue Surgery*, encompassed descriptions of different surgical procedures performed on a variety of tissue types by experts in the fields of plastic surgery, orthopedic surgery, hand surgery, esthetic surgery, and general surgery. The twelve chapters are arranged so that a direct link exists between the recently established procedures and alternative surgical options. Options that are technically possible and experimentally proven, but not applied clinically on a routine basis or even—as in the case of face transplant-not performed at this moment.

The first three chapters summarize new technical challenges in repair and restoration of function within very specialized composite tissues, such as the those of the hand or the leg. Chapter 1 summarizes the author's unique concept and experience with orthoplastic surgery as applied to limb salvage procedures. Chapter 2 introduces clinical application of composite tissue allograft transplants, such as the human hand, abdominal wall, knee, larynx, trachea, nerve, tendon muscle, and tongue. Mechanism of action of different immunosuppressive regimens and their side effects are discussed. Chapter 3 introduces versatile vascular composition of small intrinsic flaps within the hand applied for one-stage coverage of local hand defects with the advantage of early active mobilization.

Then, Chapter 4 unique describes the integrity and mobility of the subcutaneous tissue sliding system. It describes the author's personal experience and philosophy on how different tissue types in our body are interconnected and interdependent in their function. The author nicely exemplifies this relationship by presenting the unique organization of the multimicrovacuolar absorbing sliding system. The role of this system in Tendon tissue surgery, including human tendon allograft transplantation, is presented. Chapter 5 is devoted to the restoration of nerve function using novel approaches and indications for patients with diabetic neuropathy problems and patients with ankle and shoulder pain syndromes. The authors introduce their denervation technique for patient with temporomandibular joint problems.

Chapter 6 outlines minimally invasive techniques applied for peripheral nerve problems in the upper extremity. Different nerve compression syndromes are demonstrated via endoscopy , as are the results of endoscopically assisted decompression. Chapter 7 present's a sophisticated approach to perforator flap surgery and it's application to different tissues types. The author's goal is to achieve the best aesthetic outcome while minimizing donor site morbidity. Chapter 8 embarks on a search to reduce the risks of free flap failure. Methods of flap conditioning and handling are presented based on the authors' basic science experience.

Chapters 9 and 10 outline current surgical techniques applied to the most important organ in our body—the human face. In Chapter 9, techniques of face rejuvenation, with novel approaches to a variety of challenging patient populations including postbariatric surgery and HIV/AIDS patients, are presented. In contrast to traditionally accepted approaches, such as esthetic surgery, Chapter 10 presents our preparation for the most challenging procedure in tissue surgery—the human face transplantation.

Chapters 11 and 12 summarize the most current approaches to tissue engineering and stem cell based therapies. The pros and cons of clinically applying artificial tissue constructs are presented. Methods of stem cell manipulations and propagation into the different tissue types for healing and regeneration are discussed.

I hope that this book will not only introduce new methods and techniques in tissue surgery, but will also stimulate philosophical and ethical discussions on our future approaches and limitations in surgery. Maybe we are witnessing a major change in the field of tissue surgery and we will be able, in the near future, to paraphrase the Ecclesiastes aphorism that "There *is* something new under the sun."

Maria Z. Siemionow
Cleveland, Ohio

Contents

Contributors

Galip Agaoglu, MD
Department of Plastic Surgery, The
Cleveland Clinic Foundation,
Cleveland, OH, USA

Amir H. Ajar, MD
Aesthetic and Plastic Surgery Institute,
University of California, Irvine, Orange,
CA 92868, USA

Joseph Bakhach, MD
Institut Aquitain Chirurgie Plastique,
Pessac, Bordeaux, France

Phillip N. Blondeel, MD, PhD
Department of Plastic and Reconstructive
Surgery, University Hospital Gent,
Belgium

A. Lee Dellon, MD
Institute for Peripheral Nerve Surgery,
Inc., Baltimore, MD, USA

Holger Engel, MD
Department of Hand, Plastic and
Reconstructive Surgery, Burn Center,
BG-Trauma, Center Ludwigshafen,
University of Heidelberg,
Ludwigshafen, Germany

Gregory R.D. Evans, MD, FACS
The Center for Biomedical Engineering
and Aesthetic and Plastic Surgery
Institute, University of California,
Irvine, CA, USA

Günter Germann, MD, PhD
Department of Hand, Plastic and
Reconstructive Surgery, Burn Center,
BG-Trauma, Center Ludwigshafen,
University of Heidelberg,
Ludwigshafen, Germany

Jean Claude Guimberteau, MD
Institut Aquitain Chirurgie Plastique,
Pessac, Bordeaux, France

Bernd Hartmann, MD
Burn Center/Department for Plastic
Surgery, Unfallkrankenhaus Berlin,
Berlin, Germany

Reimer Hoffmann, MD
Klinik für Plastische Chirurgie und
Handchirurgie, Evangelisches
Krankenhaus Oldenburg, Oldenburg,
Germany

Markus V. Küntscher, MD, PhD
Burn Center/Department for Plastic
Surgery, Unfallkrankenhaus Berlin, Berlin,
Germany

L. Scott Levin, MD, FACS
Division of Plastic, Reconstructive
Maxillofacial and Oral Surgery, Duke
University Medical Center, Durham, NC,
USA

Christopher T. Maloney, Jr., MD
Department of Plastic Surgery,
Neurosurgery and Anatomy,
University of Arizona, Tucson, AZ,
USA

Andrea Moreira-Gonzalez, MD
Department of Plastic Surgery, The
Cleveland Clinic Foundation,
Cleveland, OH, USA

Selahattin Özmen, MD
Department of Plastic,
Reconstructive and Aesthetic Surgery,
Gazi University Faculty of Medicine,
Ankara, Turkey

Maria Z. Siemionow, MD, PhD, DSc
Department of Plastic Surgery, The
Cleveland Clinic Foundation, Cleveland
OH, USA

Sakir Unal, MD
Department of Plastic Surgery,
The Cleveland Clinic
Foundation, Cleveland, OH,
USA

James E. Zins, MD
Department of Plastic Surgery,
The Cleveland Clinic Foundation,
Cleveland, OH, USA

Orthoplastic Reconstruction of the Arms and Legs

L. Scott Levin

Introduction

By definition, a patient sustaining an open fracture in an arm or leg has a soft tissue injury, as well as a bony injury. These two injuries are inextricably linked. Since the days of Hippocrates, fractures have been stabilized by using splints or external fixators, and soft tissue injuries have been treated with various potions and salves. Techniques for proper limb alignment and soft tissue as well as fracture healing have been the subject of medicine throughout the modern era.

The history of medicine from the 16th century to the middle of the 19th century allows us to introduce the concepts of orthopaedic, plastic, and orthoplastic surgery. Individuals such as Ambroise Paré, Gaspar Tagliacozzi, Baron Guillaume Dupuytren, Alfred Louis Velpau, and Jean-François Malgaigne were master surgeons and are the founding fathers of these respected specialties.

Surgical specialties developed at the conclusion of the 19th century. Modern plastic surgery has its roots in the trenches of World War I and so is about 100 years old. Probably the first modern orthopaedic plastic collaboration was between Sir W. Arbuthnot Lane and Sir Harold Gilles. In 1919, Lane, an orthopaedic surgeon, wrote the preface for Gilles's textbook, and so began the modern era of "orthoplastic surgery."

The development of reconstructive microsurgery allowed modern orthoplastic surgery to develop. In 1960, Jacobsen and Suarez introduced the operating microscope to aid in suturing small vessels. In 1968, Tamai reported the first successful digital replantation. Other microsurgical successes evolved in the later part of the 1960s. Composite transfers of vascularized tissue became commonplace in the 1980s, with an explosion of techniques, flaps, and the popularization of microvascular surgery, not just to treat traumatic injuries of the hand and for replantation, but also for elective reconstructive surgery.[1] Refinements continued to take place, including flap preexpansion, prefabrication, and modification of tissue transfers in the 1990s.[2,3] In the later part of the 20th century, government agencies, surgical societies, and insurance companies began to ask for "outcome data," such as cost-effectiveness studies and patient-satisfaction studies to determine whether complex microsurgical procedures actually improve quality of life.[4,5]

Orthoplastic Surgery

Orthoplastic surgery as we define it is "the principles and practices of both specialties orthopaedic and plastic surgery applied to a clinical problem, either by a single provider, or teams of providers working in concert for the benefit of the patient."[5,6,7]

More than 37 years after Tamai's report that generated interest from surgeons around the world, care of the mutilated hand with microsurgical technique is standard practice.

The training of orthopaedic surgeons has shifted gradually toward performing microsurgery, whereas traditionally, mainly plastic surgeons have done microsurgery, depending on nationality. Hand and microvascular fellowships may or may not adequately prepare young surgeons to perform the full spectrum of reconstructive microsurgery, which is vitally important in orthoplastic reconstruction.

Over the past 50 years, burn care, aesthetic surgery, craniofacial surgery, and hand surgery have all become subspecialties of plastic surgery. Similarly, orthopaedic specialization has stimulated the development of separate societies concentrating on pediatric orthopaedics, trauma, musculoskeletal oncology, and hand surgery. Orthopaedics is a specialty that mainly concentrates on functional biomechanics, bone, and joints. Plastic surgery is a specialty that concentrates on aesthetics, form, and soft tissue reconstruction. The blending of these two specialties, "orthoplastic surgery," simultaneously applies the principles and practices of both specialties to clinical problems.

Historically, process-based outcome analyses, such as healing, range of motion, biomechanics, and flap success were common. Now, more emphasis is placed on patient-based outcomes as they relate to factors such as pain, functional outcome, satisfaction, and quality of life. When the outcomes movement began, the challenge was to demonstrate that this highly variable and very expensive and complicated surgery for limb salvage (orthoplastic surgery) was cost-effective and could make patients better. According to Keller, in the *Journal of the Academy of Orthopaedic Surgeons* in 1990, if surgeons cannot demonstrate this cost-effectiveness, their services could no longer be paid for![8,9]

Limb Salvage

We have learned a great deal about limb salvage compared to immediate amputation in the injured leg. We have clear indicators based on clinical assessment and scoring systems that we can share with patients before we amputate. For example, a limb that has multiple comminutions, or an elderly patient with a disruptive posterior tibial nerve, or an ipsilateral crush to the tibia and foot, cannot be salvaged (Figure 1-1). Patients that have protracted periods of ischemia with nerve disruption also make limb salvage unfeasible. We must avoid the triumph of "technology over reason." A clear understanding is needed of the prosthetic alternatives for amputees, particularly as they relate to the new technologies, such as carbon fiber, pilons, energy-absorbing ankle articulations, and special materials that allow the prosthesis to be coupled comfortably to the extremity and that will remain durable. The use of prostheses, such as the myoelectric prosthesis and the "Utah arm" for patients undergoing shoulder disarticulation

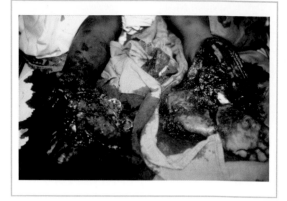

Figure 1-1. Flailed bilateral lower extremities not amenable to salvage.

injuries or tumors to the arm, are important to appreciate as alternatives to limb salvage (Figure 1-2).[10,11,12]

Orthoplastic surgery can be categorized into procedures for trauma, tumor, and septic conditions, in both the arm and leg. In addition to understanding the indications for amputations and the alternatives to limb salvage, such as a prosthesis, the modern orthopaedic surgeon should understand that there are techniques, based on biomechanics and soft tissue reconstruction, that enable the potential amputee to have a better functional residual limb.[13] These techniques include island pedicle or free flaps and fillet flaps to preserve not only sensibility but leg coverage. For example, a patient with a severe crush injury to the tibia but with a normal foot and a normal knee may require resurfacing or knee joint preservation or that the foot be filleted as an island pedicle flap or even as a free flap to provide below-knee coverage (Figure 1-3). The concept of fillet flap classifications, indications, and analysis of clinical value has been well described by Germann and others from Germany. Other examples of soft tissue augmentation of an amputation are the patient with a hip disarticulation and the patient with a midfoot amputation that can be effectively and more functionally rehabilitated with a better soft tissue envelope, often using microsurgical techniques (Figure 1-4).[14,15]

The greatest advances in orthoplastic surgery have been in the domains of trauma, tumor, and septic reconstruction. In the arm, microsurgical revascularization, rigid stabilization, and soft tissue reconstruction are common techniques for limb salvage.[16–22] In addition, we are now

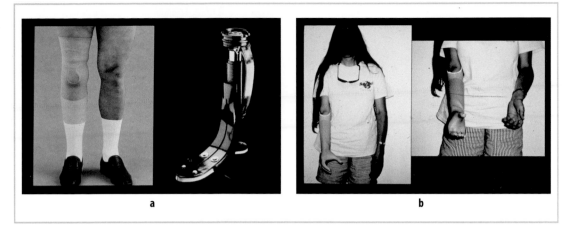

Figure 1-2. **a**) Standard below-knee prosthesis on the left, an energy-absorbing ankle on the left. **b**) An upper extremity myoelectric prosthesis.

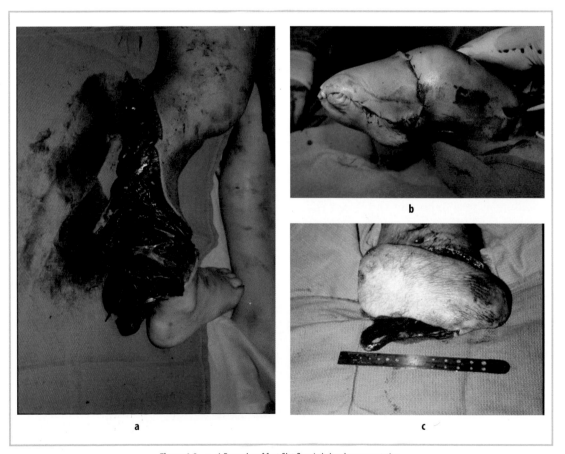

Figure 1-3. **a–c**) Examples of foot filet flaps in below-knee amputation.

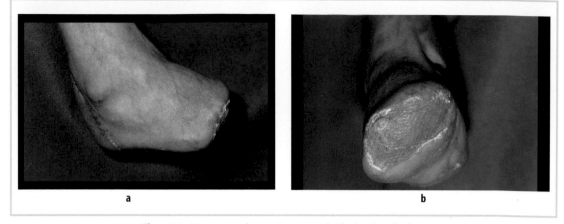

a   b

Figure 1-4. A transmetatarsal amputation augmented with a lateral arm free flap.

concentrating on the aesthetic aspects of post-traumatic reconstruction; and techniques, such as endoscopic tissue expansion, can be applied to the traumatized limb, not only to release contractures but to resurface the limb for a more aesthetically and psychologically pleasing result (Figure 1-5).[22–28]

One of the pioneers of modern orthoplastic surgery is Marco Godina, who introduced several important concepts of limb salvage. First was the concept of radical necrectomy, in which all nonviable tissue is resected and then immediately covered, such as one would do in tumor surgery with microsurgical reconstruction. Second, the concept of one-stage reconstruction, in which bony and soft tissue for coverage and function are improved to the extent possible in a single procedure, is very important and is now widely practiced (Figure 1-6).[29]

In reconstructing the arm after tumor resection, orthoplastic surgery integrates concepts from reconstructive plastic surgery into orthopaedic oncology. For example, in a child with a chondrosarcoma in the humerus that requires intercalary humeral reconstruction, the techniques related to tumor removal, fixation, vascularized bone grafting, and functional rehabilitation are all important and must be coordinated.

One of the great tools in orthoplastic surgery is the use of vascularized bone tissue, specifically the fibula.[30–34] The use of the fibula has undergone an evolution of design, beginning with transplantation of vascularized bone only (Figure 1-7). In the 1980s and 1990s the popularity of the peroneal system that can carry skin, muscle, and even innervated tissue has enjoyed popularity. An example of this reconstruction is the osteocutaneous fibula graft for treating complex forearm injuries.[30]

One should understand the reconstructive ladder as it relates to the legs in trauma, tumor, and sepsis. The proximal third of the leg, while well suited for transfers of the gastrocnemius muscle to repair relatively small anterior defects, often requires free tissue transfer for closure. One of the principles of orthoplastic surgery when dealing with a traumatic lower extremity lesion is to establish guidelines for treating bone and soft tissue early in the patient's course, preferably the night of injury. The choice of stabilization (provisional or definitive) or the choice of coverage once an extremity is deemed salvageable (planned bony reconstruction or bone grafting or tendon transfers) should all be coordinated, and a treatment plan should be defined so that expeditious care of the patient can be provided.

Just as microsurgery has had a great impact on orthoplastic surgery, thin-wire fixation (the Ilizarov technique) has had a profound influence on lower extremity and some upper extremity reconstructions.[35] The ability to do distraction osteogenesis and angular correction of bony deformities and juxta-articular deformities has greatly advanced limb salvage by providing functioning extremities. Thin-wire fixation is a very powerful tool that, when combined with microsurgery, can serve well the needs of injury repair and elective reconstruction of the lower extremity (Figure 1-8).

Examples of lower-extremity salvage include the use of the Ilizarov technique to temporarily stabilize an extremity. Soft tissue work can be done around the frame, either with local or pedicle flaps. Then the distraction or conventional bone grafting with the Ilizarov frame can be performed. In the leg, as well as in the arm, the osteocutaneous fibula can provide up to 20 cm of intercalary vascularized bone for femoral or tibia reconstruction. The fibula is well

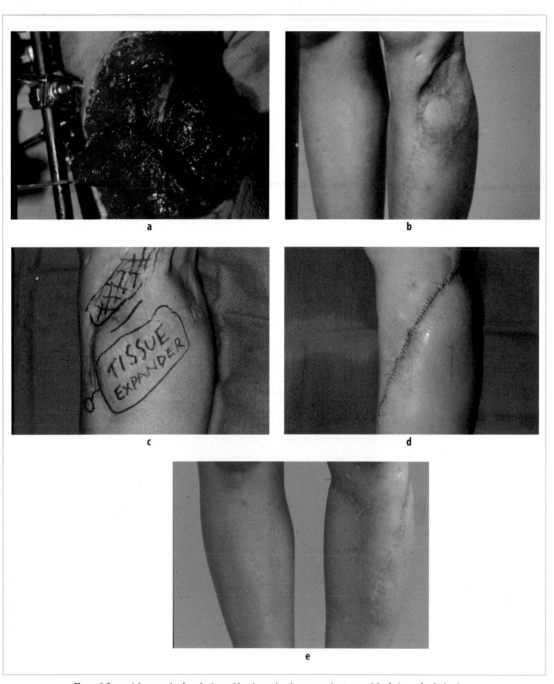

Figure 1-5. a–e) An example of aesthetic considerations using tissue expansion to remodel soft tissue after limb salvage.

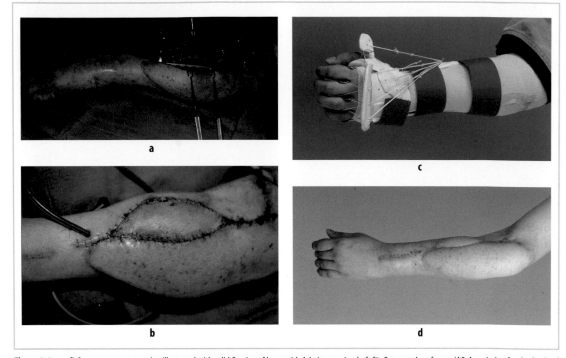

Figure 1-6. a–d) One-stage reconstruction illustrated with solid fixation of bone with Arbeitsgemeinschaft für Osteosynthesefragen (AO, Association for the Study of Osteosynthesis) principles and free tissue transfer combined.

suited for repairing large defects related to trauma or osteomyelitis in the leg. In the femur, our preference is to fold the fibula in half, to increase the cross-sectional area that mimics the diameter of the femur.

The evolution of fasciocutaneous flaps, popularized by Masquelet and based on angiosomes and perforating vessels, has added greatly to the armamentarium of soft tissue reconstructive techniques that have allowed lower limb salvage in cases where salvage was formerly not possible.[36-39]

Tumor repair in the lower limb has been enhanced by the orthoplastic approach. The use of simultaneous free flaps with tumor extirpation and allografts, as well as the Ilizarov

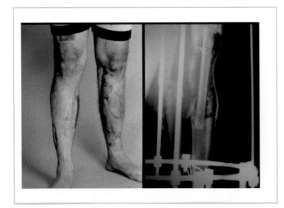

Figure 1-7. The osteocutaneous fibula in lower extremity tibia reconstruction.

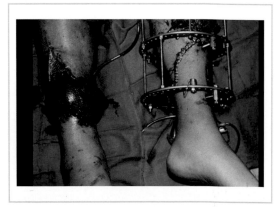

Figure 1-8. The use of external ring fixation combined with soft tissue reconstruction.

technique, has salvaged limbs that would have previously been amputated. Aesthetic considerations in the leg, as well as in the arm, can be served by tissue expansion.

Other Applications of Orthoplastic Surgery

One of the areas in orthoplastic surgery that deserves comment is osteomyelitis.[40,41] Any patient who experiences suppuration has the right to ask the surgeon to explain how it occurred. This right was pointed out by Carrel in 1918 and is still true today. Cierney and Mader classify adult osteomyelitis by anatomical type and physiological class. The anatomic types are medullary, superficial, localized, and diffuse. The physiologic classes are normal, compromised, and treatment-deferred. A clinical stage is produced by combining anatomic type with physiological class. Based on this staging

process, as in tumor surgery, the treatment outcomes for long-standing osteomyelitis can be predicted.[42]

The treatment algorithm involves the co-operation of both the soft-tissue and bone surgeons. First, radical necrectomy and sequestrectomy is performed on all nonviable tissue and implants. A healthy wound and healthy bone are then established. This process often involves removing implants; creating another stable construct, such as use of the Ilizarov or external fixation; treating dead space with soft tissue techniques, such as free flaps; and subsequently reconstructing the bone (Figure 1-9). Hyperbaric oxygen is not important in treating osteomyelitis, its current role in extremity salvage being to augment the production of granulation tissue so that any threatened dysvascular limbs of diabetic patients that are not candidates for microreconstruction or macroreconstruction can be resurfaced with skin grafts.[43,44]

Some patients undergo attempted limb salvage with proper planning and execution,

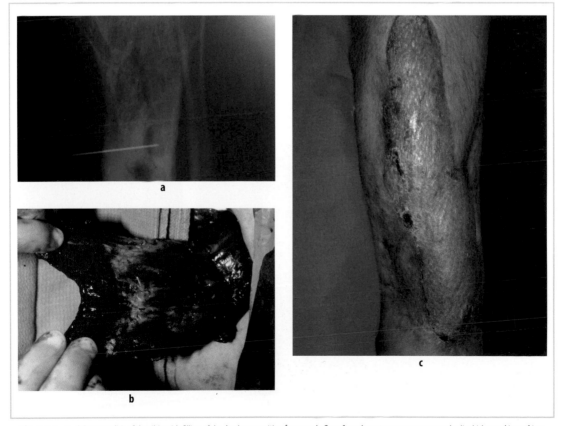

Figure 1-9. a–c) Osteomyelitis of the tibia with filling of the dead space with a free muscle flap after adequate sequestrectomy and split-thickness skin grafting.

only to result in failure as a result of chronic sepsis, intractable pain, or lack of patient desire to continue the salvage procedures. In cases where complex reconstruction has been undertaken to save threatened limbs, a contract should be made with the patient and the family indicating that if the limb cannot be saved by a certain date, amputation should be performed.

Limb salvage in patients with diabetes is especially challenging, in that a high percentage of diabetics experience neuropathy and structural changes caused by neuropathic changes in the foot, resulting in abnormal stress to the foot and leading to ulceration and skin breakdown.[45] This process often results in deep infections in the bone and soft tissue, and because diabetes inhibits healing, these infections are often resistant to conventional treatment. The first determination for limb salvage in a diabetic patient is to determine inflow, a fact often overlooked by primary care providers and even by orthopedists. Often, just simple stenting or vascular bypass procedures can augment blood flow to the limb, resulting in healing or promoting wound beds suitable for simple solutions, such as skin grafts or local flaps.[46,47] If large areas of tissue are destroyed, resulting in dead space, or if large areas need resurfacing, free tissue transfers can be considered, in conjunction with or after vascular bypass procedures.[48] The amputation rate of limbs in diabetics can be as high as 50% at 5 years; thus, all attempts should be made to salvage them.[49]

The Future of Orthoplastic Surgery

The future of orthoplastic surgery will be based on the possibility of tissue transplantation. Short of this, the use of bone allografts combined with soft tissue reconstructive techniques have been effective in salvaging limbs. Other orthoplastic domains include reconstructing the mandible with rigid fixation and vascularized bone grafts. This reconstruction problem is similar to that created by osteomyelitis in the extremities. Often radiation-induced osteonecrosis, or tumors with localized skin infection, require tumor extirpation, tissue débridement, mandibular stabilization, and soft tissue coverage. These procedures can be done as they are in the extremities.

Another domain of orthoplastic surgery that has been unrealized is the need for orthoplastic surgery of the chest wall.[50] Although soft tissue procedures are designed to treat mediastinitis and to help reconstruct the chest wall, structural instabilities, such as sternal nonunion and chronic pain based on sternal instability, can be treated with devices such as custom plates (Figure 1-10).

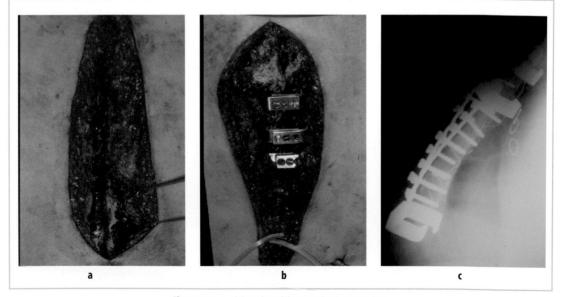

a   b   c

Figure 1-10. a–c) Sternal instability treated with custom plates.

Conclusion

Minimally invasive orthoplastic surgery has been well developed. Current techniques for tissue expansion are related to balloon-assisted endoscopic tissue expansion.[51] Free-flap prefabrication using endoscopic placement of tissue expanders has been well established and reduces the time needed for complex limb reconstruction. With minimally invasive surgery and other technologies, technologies in search of surgical procedures will not sell and be helpful. The future of orthoplastic surgery is further integration with concepts in soft tissue and bone technology and further development of limb salvage and reconstruction.

References

1. Levin LS, Condit DR. Combined injuries: soft tissue management. Clin Orthop Rel Res. 1996;(327):172–181.
2. Wang H, Erdmann D, Fletcher, Levin LS. Anterolateral thigh flap technique in hand and upper extremity reconstruction. Techniq Hand Upper Extrem Surg. 2004;8(4):257–261.
3. Levin LS, Serafin D. Plantar skin coverage. Prob Plast Reconstr Surg. 1991;1(1):156–184.
4. Keller RB, Soule DN, Wennberg JE, Hanley DF. Dealing with geographic variations in the use of hospitals: the experience of the Maine Medical Assessment Foundation Orthopaedic Study Group. J Bone Joint Surg Am. 1990;72:1286–1293.
5. Levin LS. The reconstructive ladder –an orthoplastic approach. Orthop Clin North Am. 1993;24(3):393–409.
6. Levin LS. Orthoplastic management of the wrist: an introduction. Prob Plast Reconstr Surg. 1992;2(2):141–143.
7. Levin LS. Orthoplastic reconstruction of the hand. Cur Opin Orthop. 1993;4(1):10–13.
8. Allen DM, Hey LA, Heinz TR, Golal R, Levin LS. Development and implementation of an extremity free-tissue transfer database. J Reconstr Microsurg. 1997;13(7):475–485; discussion 486–487.
9. Heinz T, Cowper P, Levin LS. Microsurgery costs and outcome. Plast Reconstr Surg. 1999;104(1):89–96.
10. Gupta A, Shatford R, Wolff TW, Tsai TW, Scheker L, Levin LS. Treatment of the severely injured upper extremity. Instr Course Lect. 2000;49:377–396; Kleinert, Christine M. Institute for Hand & Microsurgery, Louisville, KY, USA.
11. Erdmann D, Lee B, Roberts CD, Levin LS. Management of lawnmower injuries to the lower extremity in children and adolescents. Ann Plast Surg. 2000;45:595–600.
12. Levin LS. Soft tissue coverage options for ankle wounds. Foot Ankle Clin. 2001;6:853–866.
13. Erdmann D, Sundin B, Yasui K, Wong MS, Levin LS. Microsurgical free flap transfer to amputation sites: indications and results. Ann Plast Surg. 2002;48(2):167–172.
14. Levin LS, Erdmann D, Germann G. The use of fillet flaps in upper extremity reconstruction. J Am Soc Surg Hand. 2002;2(1)39–44.
15. Erdmann D, Sundin BM, Wong MS, Levin LS. Microsurgical free flap transfer to amputation sites: indications and results. Ann Plast Surg. 2002;48:167–172.
16. Levin LS, Goldner RD, Urbaniak JR, Nunley JA, Hardaker WT. Management of severe musculoskeletal injuries of the upper extremity. J Orthop Trauma. 1990;4(4):432–440.
17. Desai SS, Chuang DC, Levin LS. Microsurgical reconstruction of the extensor mechanism. Hand Clin. 1995;11(3):471–482.
18. Levin LS, Hellor L. Lower extremity microsurgical reconstruction. Plast Reconstr Surg. 2001;108(4):1029.
19. Levin LS, Zenn MR. Microsurgical reconstruction of the lower extremity. Semin Surg Oncol. 2000;19(3):272–281.
20. Heitmann C, Guerra A, Metzinger SW, Levin LS, Allen RJ. The thoracodorsal artery perforator (TDAP) flap: anatomical basis and clinical application. Ann Plast Surg. 2003;51:23–29.
21. Levin LS. Controversies and perils: beware of the traumatized gastrocnemius. Techniq Orthop. 1995;10(2):152.
22. Levin LS, Rehnke R, Eubanks S. Endoscopic surgery of the upper extremity. Hand Clinics. February 1995;11(1):59–70.
23. Lin CH, Levin LS. Free flap expansion using balloon-assisted endoscopic technique. Microsurgery. 1996;17(6):330–336.
24. Van Buskirk ER, Rehnke RD, Montgomer RL, Eubanks S, Ferraro FJ, Levin LS. Endoscopic harvest of the latissimus dorsi muscle using the balloon dissection technique. Plast Reconstr Surg. 1997;99(3):899–903; discussion, 904–905.
25. Ip TY, Aponte R, Koger KE, Germann G, Zobrist R, Levin LS. Use of balloon dissector in minimally invasive aesthetic and reconstructive surgery. Ann Plast Surg. 1998;40(3):205–213.
26. Lin CH, Wei FC, Levin LS, Chen MC. Donor-site morbidity comparison between endoscopically assisted and traditional harvest of free latissimus dorsi muscle flap. Plast Reconstr Surg. 1999;104(4):823.
27. Heinz T, Levin LS. Aesthetic considerations after limb trauma. Techniq Orthp. 1995;10(2):94–103.
28. Levin LS, Aponte R, Germann G. Endoscopic tissue expansion of the upper extremity. Op Techniq Plast Reconstr Surg. 1997;4(1):24–30.
29. Levin LS, Erdmann DE. Primary and secondary microvascular reconstruction of the upper extremity. Hand Clin. 2001;17(3):447–455.
30. Jupiter JB, Gerhard HJ, Guerrero J, Nunley JA, Levin LS. Treatment of segmental defects of the radius with use of the vascularized osteoseptocutaneous fibular autogenous Graft. J Bone Joint Surg. 1997;79(4):542–550.
31. Lin CH, Wei FC, Levin LS, Su JI, Fan KF, Yeh W, et al. Free composite serratus anterior and rip flaps for tibial composite bone and soft-tissue defect. Plast Reconstr Surg. 1997;99(6):1656–1665.
32. Heitmann C, Erdmann D, Levin LS. Treatment of segmental defects of the humerus with the use of osteoseptocutaneous fibula graft. J Bone Joint Surg. 2002;84(12):2216–2223.

33. Erdmann D, Bergqvist GEO, Levin LS. Ipsilateral free fibula transfer for reconstruction of a segmental femoral-shaft defect. *Brit J Plast Surg.* 2002;55: 675–677.

34. Levin LS, Heitmann C, Khan F. Vasculature of the peroneal artery: an anatomic study focused on the perforator vessels. *J Reconstr Microsurg.* 2003;19(3):157–162.

35. Levin LS. Combined free tissue transplantation and Ilizarov for lower extremity salvage. Young Microsurgeon's Perspective Newsletter. *Am Soc Reconstr Microsurg.* January 1996.

36. Levin LS, Aponte RL, Nunley JA. Soft-tissue coverage for the foot and ankle. *Foot Ankle Clin.* 1999;4(3): 853–866.

37. Baumeister S, Spierer R, Erdmann D, Sweis R, Levin LS, Germann G. A realistic complication analysis of 70 sural flaps in a multimorbid patient group. *Plast Reconstr Surg.* 2003;112:129–142.

38. Heitmann C, Levin LS. The orthoplastic approach in the management of the severely traumatized foot and ankle. *J Trauma.* 2003;54:379–390.

39. Levin LS. Regional flap alternatives to microsurgery in the dysvascular extremity. *Op Techniq Plast Reconstr Surg.* 1997;4(4):236–249.

40. Heitmann C, Patzakis MJ, Tetsworth K, Levin LS. Musculoskeletal sepsis: principles of treatment. *Instr Course Lect.* 2003;52:733–743.

41. Heitmann C, Higgins L, Levin LS. Treatment of deep shoulder infections with pedicled myocutaneous flaps. *J Shoulder Elbow Surg.* 2004;13(1):13–17.

42. Harvey EJ, Aponte R, Levin LS. The application of the island pedicle latissimus dorsi flap for soft tissue coverage of the elbow. *Can Plast Surg J.* 1999;(1):23–26, 1999.

43. Gates H, Levin LS, Harrelson J, Urbaniak JR. The use of hyperbaric oxygen in treatment of chronic osteomyelitis. *Orthop Trans.* 1988;12(3):524.

44. Maynor ML, Moon RE, Camporesi EM, Fawcett TA, Fracia PJ, Norfell HC, et al. Chronic osteomyelitis of the tibia: treatment with hyperbaric oxygen and autogenous microsurgical muscle transplantation. *J South Orthop Assoc.* 1998;7(1):43–57.

45. Oishi SN, Levin LS, Pederson WC. Microsurgical management of extremity wounds in diabetics with peripheral vascular disease. *Plast Reconstr Surg.* 1993;92(3): 485–492.

46. Ritter EF, Anthony JP, Levin LS, Demas CP, Klitzman B, Skarada DL, et al. Microsurgical composite tissue transplantation at difficult recipient sites facilitated by preliminary installation of vein grafts as arterviovenous loops. *J Reconstr Microsurg.* 1996;12(4):231–240.

47. Lin CH, Levin LS. The functional outcome of lower extremity fractures with vascular injury. *J Trauma.* 1999;43(3):480–485.

48. Levin LS, Nunley JA. Management of soft tissue problems associated with calcaneal fractures. *Clin Orthop Rel Res.* 1993;(290):151–156.

49. Levin LS, Barwick W, Pederson WC, Brenman S, Serafin D. Long-term follow-up of autologous tissue transplantation to the foot and ankle. *J Reconstr Microsurg.* 1991;7(3):253.

50. Hendrickson SC, Koger KE, Morea CJ, Aponte R, Smith PK, Levin LS. Sternal plating for treatment of sternal nonunion. *Ann Thorac Surg.* 1996;62(2):512–518.

51. Ip TY, Aponte R, Koger KE, Germann G, Zobrist R, Levin LS. Use of the balloon dissector in minimally invasive aesthetic and reconstructive surgery. *Ann Plast Surg.* 1998;40(3):205–213.

2

Clinical Application of Composite Tissue Allografts

Maria Z. Siemionow, Sakir Unal and Galip Agaoglu

Introduction

Composite tissue allografts (CTAs) consist of tissues derived from ectoderm and mesoderm and typically contain skin, fat, muscle, nerves, lymph nodes, bone, cartilage, ligaments, and bone marrow. Although "nonvital" to life, these tissues are structurally, functionally, and aesthetically important to patients who need functional restoration of musculoskeletal defects.

Autologous tissue is the most commonly used material for reconstructing severe burn and traumatic injuries or cancer ablation surgeries. Even when enough autologous tissue is available to reconstruct large defects, functional and aesthetic recovery is not always ideal, and multiple surgeries may be necessary. In addition, donor site morbidity can be a problem in autologous tissue grafting. Prosthetic materials are another treatment option for large defects, but they have all the major drawbacks of nonvital material. Composite tissue allografts thus have great potential for reconstructing various parts of the body.

Composite tissue is more immunogenic than transplanted solid organs. Although cartilage, ligaments, and fat have low antigenicity and bone, muscles, nerves, and vessels have moderate antigenicity, skin develops the most severe rejection because of the abundance of dendritic cells in the epidermis and dermis.[1]

Clinical Composite Tissue Allotransplants

Advances in transplantation immunology have opened discussion on the routine clinical applicability of composite tissue allografts. As of January 1, 2005, more than 50 composite tissue allograft transplants have been performed worldwide, including; hand, abdominal wall, knees, flexor tendon apparatus, nerve, larynx, skeletal muscle, tongue, and trachea (Table 2-1).

Hand Transplants

The first hand transplantation was performed before the cyclosporine era of immunosuppression in 1963.[2] The patient received steroids and azathioprine immunosuppressive treatment. The hand was rejected 3 weeks after transplantation.

Since the first successful hand transplantation in 1998, in Lyon[3], 25 transplants (6 bilateral) in 19 patients have been reported; 8 (6 patients) from China, 5 (3 patients) from France, 4 (2 patients) from Austria, 3 from Italy, 2 from the USA, 1 from Belgium, and 1 from Malaysia (Table 2-2).[4]

In September 1998, a team in Lyons, France, performed the first successful human hand allotransplant.[3] They transplanted the right hand and distal forearm from a brain-dead donor to a 48-year-old man whose own right hand and distal forearm had been amputated in a 1989 accident. The induction immunosuppressive protocol consisted initially of antithymocyte globulin (75 mg/day for 10 days), tacrolimus adjusted to maintain blood concentrations between 10 ng/mL and 15 ng/mL during the first month, mycophenolate mofetil (MMF) (2 g/day), and steroids (prednisone, 250 mg on day 1 and rapidly tapered to 20 mg/day). CD25 monoclonal antibody was given on day 26 and day 100. Maintenance therapy included tacrolimus (to maintain serum concentrations between 5 and 10 ng/mL), MMF (2 g/day), and prednisone (20 mg/day at 3 months, 15 mg/day at 6 months).[3] At 6-month follow-up, progression of motor and sensory function was satisfactory.

In January 1999, surgeons in Louisville, Kentucky, performed the first human hand

Table 2-1. Number and Type of Composite Tissue Allografts Transplanted as of January 1, 2005, Worldwide

Hand	13 unilateral, 6 bilateral
Abdominal wall	9
Knee	3 femoral diaphysis, 5 whole knee
Flexor tendon apparatus	2
Nonvascularized nerve	7
Larynx	1
Muscle	1
Tongue	1
Trachea	2

allotransplant in the United States.[5] They transplanted a donor hand to a 37-year-old man whose own left hand was lost in an accident in 1985. Postoperative immunosuppressive therapy consisted of intravenous basiliximab (20 mg on days 0 and 4), tacrolimus (target trough 15 to 20 ng/mL), MMF (1 g twice daily, plasma concentrations between 3 and 5 ng/mL), and prednisone (2 mg/kg/day tapered to 10 mg/day by 3 months). Neuromuscular function returned more rapidly in the allograft hand than it does in replanted hands, and there was less stiffness and edema.

French and Italian teams have reported the largest series of 8 hand transplants in 6 patients (4 single and 2 double transplants).[6] In these 8 hands, the time between amputation and transplant ranged from 3 to 22 years. The level of amputation in the recipients was at the wrist in 6 hands and at the distal forearm in 2. Cold ischemia time ranged from 11 to 12.5 hours. The sequence of the surgical procedure was bone fixation, revascularization with microsurgical anastomoses of at least one artery and vein, tendon repair, nerve coaptation, and skin closure. The immunosuppressive protocol included an initial induction therapy using polyclonal antibodies or anti-CD25 monoclonal antibody, tacrolimus, MMF, and prednisone. Maintenance therapy included tacrolimus (blood levels maintained between 5 and 10 ng/mL), mycophenolate mofetil (1 to 2 g/day), and prednisone (2.5 to 7.5 mg/day). In two cases, additional surgical procedures were performed. Tendons were shortened for better wrist stability in one case, and trauma to the extensor pollicis longus tendon was repaired in the other.

The rehabilitation protocol started as soon as the swelling subsided and included physiotherapy, electrostimulation, and occupational therapy; and therapy continued for up to 24 months. The mean postoperative hospital stay was 22.6 days. Two of the 6 patients restarted their previous jobs within 5 months of surgery. Another unemployed patient started to work after surgery.

At least once, every patient had signs of skin rejection, at a mean of 40 days postoperatively. Two patients had a second rejection episode at an average of 82 days postoperatively. After 18 months, discriminative sensation returned and continued to improve thereafter. Motor recovery has been good in all patients, enabling them to perform a number of daily activities, including eating, drinking, driving, shaving, phoning, and writing. Functional magnetic resonance imaging revealed progressive recovery of sensorimotor activations of the cortex for the hand area within 6 months postoperatively, indicating a good degree of cortical reintegration.[7]

The first hand transplant was re-amputated because the patient was nonadherent to physical therapy and immunosuppressive treatment. This case shows the importance of patient selection; it also demonstrates the reversibility of hand transplantation for cases with undesired complications or for patients with unsatisfactory results. Recently, one of the Chinese recipients experienced refractory rejection, which was treated with local injections of steroids. One of these injections was accidentally released into the artery, which led to graft loss.[4]

The main concern with hand transplantation, as with other CTA transplants, is the need to

Table 2-2. Cases of Hand Transplantation as of January 1, 2005, Worldwide

Date	Location	Transplant Type
1963	Ecuador	Unilateral
September 1998	Lyon (France)	Unilateral
January 1999	Louisville (KY, USA)	Unilateral
September 1999	Guangzhou (China)	Unilateral
September 1999	Guangzhou (China)	Unilateral
January 2000	Lyon (France)	Bilateral
January 2000	Guangxi (China)	Unilateral
January 2000	Guangxi (China)	Unilateral
March 2000	Innsbruck (Austria)	Bilateral
May 2000	Kuala Lumpur (Malaysia)	Unilateral
October 2000	Guangzhou (China)	Bilateral
August 2000	Monza (Italy)	Unilateral
January 2001	Harping (China)	Bilateral
February 2001	Louisville (KY, USA)	Unilateral
October 2001	Monza (Italy)	Unilateral
June 2002	Brussels (Belgium)	Unilateral
November 2002	Milan (Italy)	Unilateral
February 2003	Innsbruck (Austria)	Bilateral
May 2003	Lyon (France)	Bilateral
Total	**19 patients**	**25 hands**

expose patients to lifelong immunosuppression. Immunosuppressive protocols used in hand transplants are almost similar to those used in solid organ transplants and usually include a combination of tacrolimus, MMF, and prednisone for induction therapy; and tacrolimus and MMF or tacrolimus and prednisone for maintenance therapy. Antithymocyte globulin (ATG) and anti-CD25 monoclonal antibody were used for induction therapy in 2 patients.[8] Episodes of rejection were treated with an increase in prednisone and with topical applications of steroids and tacrolimus.

The most commonly reported complications are transient hyperglycemia, which was treated with insulin; viral and fungal infections, treated with antiviral and antifungal agents; and Cushing syndrome. High serum creatinine, anemia, and transient hypertension and avascular bone necrosis were among other side effects of immunosuppressive agents. These complications were treated by reducing the dosage of immunosuppressive drugs.[4,0]

The Carroll test was used to evaluate the functional recovery of hand transplants. On a scale of 0 to 99, with 99 being the best result, scores greater than 85 are excellent, scores between 74 and 85 are good, scores between 51 and 84 are fair, and scores less than 51 are poor. The average score for the first 4 (2 from USA and 2 from China) transplants was 63. This average compares to the Carroll score of 70 for the best replantations.[4,8]

Hand transplantations have had successful clinical results, and no evidence of chimerism has been found in the transplanted hands so far.

Abdominal Wall Transplants

Levi et al. reported 9 cadaveric abdominal wall composite allograft transplants in 8 patients.[9] The abdominal wall composite allograft included one or both rectus abdominis muscles, fascia, subcutaneous tissue, and skin. The blood supply was derived from the donor inferior epigastric vessels, left in continuity with the larger femoral and iliac vessels. In the recipient, the abdominal wall graft vessels were anastomosed to the common iliac artery and vein. The surface area of coverage provided by the abdominal wall graft ranged from $150 \, cm^2$ to $500 \, cm^2$. All transplants were carried out without HLA (human leukocyte antigens) matching. Seven of 8 patients received

ABO-identical grafts. One patient with blood type A received an ABO-identical multivisceral graft, followed 6 days later with a blood type O abdominal wall graft from a second donor. Recipients received either an isolated small-bowel or multivisceral allografts. Seven patients received the anti-CD52 monoclonal antibody alemtuzumab (0.3 mg/kg IV) immediately before surgery and at postoperative days 3 and 7. Maintenance immunosuppression was based on tacrolimus (10 µ/L) without corticosteroids. One patient received daclizumab as an induction agent, instead of alemtuzumab. Intravenous corticosteroids were used to treat rejection. Of 8 patients, 6 are alive, and 5 have functioning, viable abdominal wall composite grafts. The skin of the abdominal wall was mildly rejected in 2 patients, but they completely recovered with corticosteroid therapy. Transplantation of the abdominal wall was essential for coverage of the transplanted visceral allografts and patient's survival.

Knee Transplants

In 1994, Hoffman and Kirschner used vascularized bone allotransplantations to treat the sequela of tumors and trauma of the legs.[10] Three patients received a femoral diaphysis, and 5 patients received the whole knee joint with its extensor system. All patients received allotransplants from ABO-matched and HLA-mismatched donors.

Recipients received cyclosporine A (CsA; 1.5 mg/kg IV), azathioprine (1.5 mg/kg IV), ATG (4 mg/kg IV), and methylprednisolone (250 mg) for immunosuppression for 3 days, after which CsA was reduced to 6.0 mg/kg PO and azathioprine to 3.0 mg/kg PO. After 6 months, azathioprine was withdrawn, and patients were kept on CsA alone until bone consolidation of the two osteotomies was complete. In the femur recipients, immunosuppressive therapy was stopped 2 years after surgery.

After 2 to 5 years of follow-up, the allograft was favorably integrated in 4 patients, and the range of motion of the knee was satisfactory.[8,11] However, 1 femur allograft and 3 knee allografts were replaced with autografts or prosthetics because of infection. On the basis of this preliminary study and discussions at the Second International Symposium on CTA Transplantation in Louisville, the following conclusions were reached: 1) vascularized femoral diaphysis transplantation and knee joint allografts should be considered the last choice of treatment; 2) intramedullary osteosynthesis appears to offer better results than external fixation or plate osteosynthesis; 3) cyclosporine A and azathioprine immunosuppression protocols have no adverse impact on bone healing, but they did not suppress acute or chronic episodes of rejection; 4) synovial membranes, as the primary target of rejection, require lifelong immunosuppression; 5) vascularized bone allografts, as low-flow organs, may have a high risk of thrombosis and necrosis; 6) more studies are required to determine optimal cold ischemia time and optimal storing temperature for bone grafts; 7) neuropathic arthropathy could occur as a result of bone and joint denervation; and 8) because the procedure is complex, it should be performed in selected centers by surgeons with adequate backgrounds and technical skills.

Flexor Tendon Apparatus Transplants

In 1988 and 1989, Guimberteau et al. reported 2 vascularized digital flexor tendon apparatus allotransplants.[12] Both patients had been operated on several times with unsatisfactory results. One allograft was from a living nonrelated donor whose little finger had to be amputated to provide the requisite tissues. The blood group and the HLA of donor and recipient were not identical. Mixed lymphocyte reaction was nonreactive. The second allograft was from a cadaver donor. The ABO group was identical, and there was no major HLA incompatibility between the donor and recipient. The tendon allografts in both cases were based on the ulnar vessels. After inset of the grafts, the ulnar arteries of the donor and the recipient were anastomosed. Venous anastomoses were performed between the ulnar veins in the living nonrelated donor and between the donor ulnar vein and the superficial forearm vein in the second allograft.

Both patients received CsA monotherapy, 7 mg, for only 6 months because of the low antigenicity of the tendon structures. The grafts were accepted without rejection, and the vessels remained patent. After 1 year, active flexion of fingers in both patients had improved. In the living nonrelated tendon allograft, the range of motion was improved from none preoperatively to 75° with

an extension deficit of 15° in the proximal interphalangeal joint and to 50° in the distal interphalangeal joint, with an extension deficit of 45°. There was no change in the range of motion in the metacarpophalangeal joint. In the second allograft, the range of motion improved from none preoperatively to 80° in the proximal interphalangeal joint, with no extension deficit, and to 55° in the distal interphalangeal joint, with an extension deficit of 35°.

Nerve Transplants

Mackinnon et al.'s series of 7 patients with peripheral nerve allografts is the only reported series with long follow-up.[13] Of 7 allografts, 4 were used in the arms and 3 in the legs. All patients had traumatic injuries of their arms or legs and massive peripheral nerve deficits that could not be reconstructed by conventional means. The grafts were harvested from the limbs of cadaver donors and were preserved in cold ischemia at 5°C for 7 days before implantation. This delay was planned to decrease the immunogenicity of the transplant by decreasing the expression of MHC (major histocompatibility complex) on the surface of cells. Mackinnon et al. showed that 1 week of cold preservation does not decrease the number of viable donor Schwann cells but does reduce the expression of major histocompatibility complex class II molecules critical to T-cell immunoactivation.[14,15] In a sheep model, increasing the length of cold preservation revealed low allograft immunogenicity, as measured by decreased and altered lymphocytic infiltration into the nerve allografts.[16]

The length of the nerve defect was 12 cm to 37 cm. Because small-diameter nerve allografts are better vascularized than large nerve allografts, depending on the proximal nerve stump diameter, 3 to 10 cables were used. The mean total length of the allograft used in one patient was 190 cm (range: 72 to 350 cm). The first 5 patients received CsA (200 to 300 ng/mL blood levels), azathioprine (1 to 1.5 mg/kg/day), and prednisone (initially 0.25 to 0.5 mg/kg/day and tapered off over 4 to 8 weeks). Tacrolimus (5 to 15 ng/mL/blood levels) replaced CsA for the last 2 patients. Immunosuppressive therapy was maintained for 6 months after finding evidence of nerve regeneration (Tinel's sign) distal to the graft. The mean duration of immunosuppression was 18 months (range: 12 to 26 months). Rejection in one patient led to graft loss 4 months after transplantation. The 6 other patients recovered distal sensibility. All recovered sensation, and 3 recovered motor abilities. None of the patients showed any evidence of deterioration of nerve function after the withdrawal of immunosuppressive therapy.[13]

Larynx Transplants

In 1998, Strome et al. performed the first successful larynx transplantation.[17,18] The recipient was a 40-year-old aphonic male who had sustained a crush injury to his larynx 20 years before. The donor was a 40-year-old male who had died from a ruptured cerebral aneurysm. Transplanted complex included the donor's larynx, thyroid gland, parathyroid glands, 5 rings of trachea, and most of the donor's pharynx, to widen the recipient's pharynx. In the recipient, arterial anastomoses were performed to the superior thyroid arteries bilaterally, and venous anastomoses were performed to the common facial vein on the right side and to the internal jugular vein on the left side. The patient's right recurrent laryngeal nerve and both superior laryngeal nerves were coapted to the donor's nerves.

The patient received muromonab-CD3 (5 mg/day), cyclosporine A (500 mg/day), methylprednisolone (50 mg/day, with the dose decreased to 20 mg/day by postoperative day 4), and MMF (1 g twice daily) during the first week after surgery. Subsequently, the patient received cyclosporine, MMF, and prednisone in progressively decreasing doses. Six months after transplantation, the patient's blood pressure and serum creatinine were elevated and were treated by additional antihypertensive drugs and by decreasing the CsA dose. At 15 months, one episode of rejection was observed and manifested by reduction in the quality of the voice and ultimately aphonia. The larynx returned to normal within 3 days of treatment with high doses of prednisone. Then, CsA was replaced with tacrolimus.

The patient's phonation improved steadily and became stable at normal levels 16 months after transplantation. At 16 months, the pitch of the voice changed and became more natural. At 36 months, the speech of the patient was almost normal. The patient obtained efficient deglutition after 3 months. Currently, the patient talks with a natural and intelligible voice, feeds himself without aspiration, and has an improved sense of taste and smell.[18] Four years after transplantation, laryngeal electromyography revealed re-innervation of the laryngeal muscle.[19]

Potential candidates for laryngeal transplantation include aphonic patients with laryngeal trauma, large benign chondromas, or laryngeal carcinoma who are cancer-free for 5 years.

Muscle Transplants

In 1998, vascularized skeletal muscle allografting was done to cover a large defect in the scalp of a renal transplant patient who was on chronic immunosuppressive therapy (CsA and prednisone).[20] After the second cadaveric renal transplant, squamous cell carcinoma developed in the scalp. The tumor was excised, and the defect was reconstructed with a cadaveric vascularized rectus femoris muscle flap. The patient received methylprednisolone, 1 g, and rabbit antithymocyte globulin, 1.5 mg/kg IV, before revascularization. He was returned immediately to his baseline immunosuppressive regimen of prednisone and CsA. A muscle biopsy 2 weeks after transplant revealed perivascular lymphocytic infiltration, and MMF (1000 mg PO b.i.d.) was administered, and the dose of CsA was increased. At 18 weeks, MMF was stopped, and the patient was kept on chronic CsA and prednisone. This patient is still under immunosuppression for kidney transplant with no reported complications.

Tongue Transplants

On July 19, 2003, the world's first tongue transplantation was performed, in a patient with tongue cancer.[21] No report on the immunosuppression protocol was given for this procedure. The patient was discharged from the hospital 1 month after surgery with a tracheostomy and a gastrostomy. After 8 months, there was no sign of rejection, and the patient was able to swallow his saliva and some fluids. Although tongue transplant represents a promising alternative for conventional tongue reconstruction, it is unlikely to restore a sense of taste. Longer follow-up is needed to address this issue.

Trachea Transplants

Transplantation of the human trachea remains an unsolved technical problem because the trachea lacks of a well-defined blood supply. Although a number of experimental approaches have been studied to solve this problem,[22] only a few attempts to transplant the trachea in humans have been reported. In 1979, Rose et al. reported a heterotopic implantation by wrapping the trachea in the sternocleidomastoid muscle.[23] Three weeks later, orthotopic implantation was performed, accompanied by a vascularized muscular section from the sternocleidomastoid. After 9 weeks, and without immunosuppression protocol, no signs of rejection or ischemia were apparent. However, no further information on the long-term results is available.

Levashov and colleagues reported the second case of human tracheal transplantation in 1993.[24] A 24-year-old woman with idiopathic fibrosing mediastinitis affecting the thoracic segment of the trachea received an allograft replacement of the distal trachea wrapped with omentum. Although the patient was on cyclosporine A immunosuppression, early rejection after 10 days was treated by increasing the dose of immunosuppression. The functional outcome after 2 months of transplantation was good. However, progressive stenosis eventually required permanent stenting of the trachea.

In 2004, Klepetko et al. reported heterotopic tracheal transplantation with omentum wrapping in the abdomen.[25] A 57-year-old patient with chronic obstructive pulmonary disease and low-segment tracheal stenosis was accepted for lung transplantation and 2-stage tracheal allotransplantation. During lung transplantation, the trachea was wrapped with omentum in the abdomen. Triple immunosuppressive therapy was started with intravenous cyclosporine A, MMF, and corticosteroids, and was maintained orally thereafter. Eight months after lung transplantation, 5 cm of tracheal segment was excised, and the defect was closed with no need for tracheal allograft transplantation. Therefore, the tracheal allograft was harvested and investigated completely. Hematoxylin-eosin staining revealed vital cartilage covered by respiratory epithelium. The tracheal wall was highly vascularized, indicating allograft viability without signs of rejection.

Immunosuppressive Drugs Currently Used in Composite Tissue Allograft Transplants

Currently, immunosuppressive drugs are used to induce, maintain, and treat acute episodes of graft rejection (Table 2-3). All current immunosuppressive drugs target activation of T cells, production of cytokines, clonal expansion, or a combination of all these factors (Table 2-4; Figure 2-1).[26]

Immunosuppression Induction Protocols

The aim of inducing immunosuppression after transplantation is to suppress the immune system for a short period (2 weeks) to reduce the possibility of hyperacute (within 10 days after transplant) and acute rejection (within 3 months after the transplant).[26]

Table 2-3. Immunosuppressive Therapy Regimens Used in Transplanting Composite Tissue Allografts

Transplant	Induction Therapy	Maintenance Therapy
Hand	ATG Anti-CD25 MoAb Tacrolimus MMF Basiliximab Prednisone	Tacrolimus MMF Prednisone
Abdominal wall	Anti-CD52 MoAb (alemtuzumab) Daclizumab	Tacrolimus
Vascularized bone	ATG CsA Azathioprine Prednisone	CsA Azathioprine
Nonvascularized nerve	CsA or tacrolimus Azathioprine Prednisone	CsA or tacrolimus Azathioprine Prednisone
Vascularized tendon	CsA	CsA
Nonvascularized trachea	CsA MMF	CsA MMF
Larynx	OKT3 CsA MMF	CsA or tacrolimus MMF Prednisone
Muscle	ATG	CsA Prednisone

ATG = antithymocyte globulins
MMF = mycophenolate mofetil
CsA = cyclosporine A
OKT3 = anti-CD3 antibody

Table 2-4. Immunosuppressive Drugs used in Transplanting Composite Tissue Allografts

Drug	Mechanism of Action
	Lymphocyte-Depleting Agents
Antithymocyte globulins/Antilymphocyte globulin (ATG/ALG)	Binds multiple antigens on lymphocytes and causes complement mediated lysis and opsonization
Anti-CD3 antibody (OKT3)	Blocks T-cell CD3 receptor and causes complement mediated lysis and opsonization
	Interleukin-2 Receptor Antagonists
Daclizumab	Binds Interleukin-2 receptor and down-regulates
Basiliximab	Binds Interleukin-2 receptor and down-regulates
	Cytokine Gene Expression Blockers
Steroids	Blocks the transcription of cytokine genes
	Nonspecific actions to decrease immune reactivity
	Calcineurin Inhibitors
Cyclosporine	Inhibits calcineurin, and Interleukin-2 production
Tacrolimus (FK-506)	Inhibits calcineurin, and Interleukin-2 production
	Antiproliferative Agents
Mycophenolate mofetil (MMF)	Blocks de novo purine synthesis
Azathioprine	Blocks synthesis
	TOR (Target of Rapamycin) Inhibitor
Sirolimus	Blocks IL-2–induced cell cycle progression

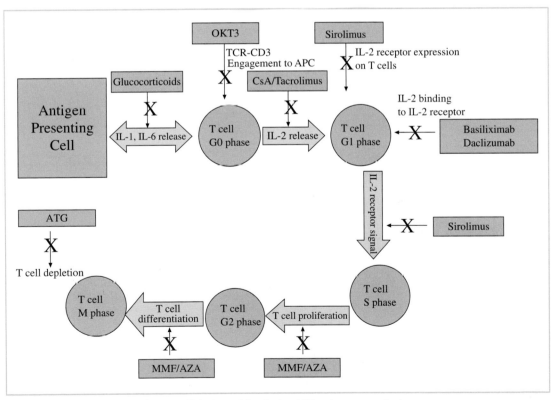

Figure 2-1. Mechanisms and sites of action of different immunosuppressive drugs

Induction protocols consist of a 7-day to 14-day course of treatment. Immunosuppressive drugs commonly used for induction therapy are polyclonal antithymocyte globulins (ATG), anti-interleukin-2 (IL-2) receptor monoclonal antibodies (daclizumab and basiliximab), and anti-CD3 monoclonal antibodies, such as OKT3.

Immunosuppression Maintenance Protocols

Maintenance drugs are used to diminish the ability of the recipient's immune system to identify and reject the transplanted tissue. Various combinations of immunosuppressants are used for maintenance therapy. Different combinations achieve a potent immunosuppressive effect with the use of low doses of individual drugs. Combinations usually aim to minimize the adverse and toxic effects of these drugs and, in the meantime, to block T-cell activation at various steps. These protocols commonly include corticosteroids combined with calcineurin inhibitors (CsA, FK-506), antiproliferative agents (azathioprine, MMF), and rapamycin inhibitors (sirolimus).

Treatment of Acute Rejection

Corticosteroids are the first choice of treatment in acute rejection episodes. In cases where corticosteroids do not suppress acute attacks of rejection, the drugs used in induction therapy (ATG and OKT3) or maintenance therapy (tacrolimus and sirolimus) can be used. Topical corticosteroids and topical tacrolimus have successfully treated rejection in recipients of composite tissue grafts.[26]

Calcineurin Inhibitors (Cyclosporine A and FK-506)

Calcineurin is a phosphatase that is important for IL-2 gene transcription and release by T cells. Phosphorylation and dephosphorylation of specific proteins help regulate cytokine production in T cells. Both CsA and tacrolimus are prodrugs; they need to form a complex with cellular proteins called "immunophilins" before exerting their effects. Cyclosporine A binds to cyclophilin, whereas tacrolimus binds to FK-binding proteins. After the drugs are bound, they render the calcineurin complex inactive, preventing subsequent gene transcription of IL-2, thereby reducing the production of IL-2, a key cytokine for T-cell expansion, and of other cytokines.[27]

Cyclosporine A is a metabolite extracted from *Trichoderma polysporum* fungus. Cyclosporine A is highly specific for T cells and inhibits the activation of both CD4+ and CD8+. The effects of CsA in suppressing IL-2 production can be reversed by discontinuing the drug. The effect of CsA in blocking IL-2 release can be increased when used in combination with corticosteroids.[26–28]

Tacrolimus (FK-506) is a metabolite of an actinomycete, *Streptomyces tsukubaensis*, and is an effective alternative to cyclosporine. The structure of tacrolimus is different from that of CsA, and the mechanism of action is similar to that of cyclosporine. In vitro, tacrolimus appears to be 100 times more potent than CsA.[29] Tacrolimus suppresses transcription of cytokines IL-2, IL-3, IL-4, IL-5, IFN-γ, and TNF-α, as well as granulocyte macrophage colony stimulating factor.[30]

Both tacrolimus and CsA have similar renal and hepatic toxicities, but they differ in other toxic side effects. Patients treated with tacrolimus have a higher incidence of diabetes mellitus but a lower incidence of hypertension, hyperlipidemia, and hirsutism.[31] Tacrolimus is more potent than CsA in enhancing peripheral nerve regeneration and is therefore commonly used in human hand transplantation.[32]

Sirolimus (TOR Inhibitor)

Sirolimus (rapamycin) is structurally similar to tacrolimus and is extracted from the actinomycete *Streptomyces hygroscopicus*. Sirolimus, like tacrolimus, binds to FK-binding protein-12, but unlike tacrolimus, it does not inhibit calcineurin phosphatase. Sirolimus blocks calcium-independent events during the G1 phase. Its immunosuppressive effect is by inhibiting TOR (target of rapamycin), which is an important enzyme in T-cell proliferation. TOR inhibitor, unlike calcineurin inhibitors, fails to interfere in the early events after T-cell activation. However, it overcomes other CsA-resistant pathways in T-cell and B-cell stimulation. Therefore, it inhibits the proliferation and maturation of B cells, which leads to extreme depression of host alloantibodies after allografting in a sensitized host.[30]

Adding sirolimus to combination regimens has allowed the dose of calcineurin inhibitors to be reduced, thus decreasing the nephrotoxicity associated with calcineurin inhibitors without decreasing graft survival.[33] The main side effects of sirolimus are hypercholesterolemia, leukopenia, and thrombocytopenia; and, unlike calcineurin inhibitors, hypertension, nephrotoxicity, and hepatotoxicity are not common.[26]

Corticosteroids

Corticosteroids are nonspecific anti-inflammatory agents that inhibit cytokine production by T cells and macrophages. In the initial phase of transplantation, they affect cytokine gene transcription and inhibit the secretion of several important cytokines, such as IL-1, IL-2, IL-6, TNF-β, and IFN-γ, which are important in inflammatory reactions.

Corticosteroids were originally used to treat acute episodes of rejection in patients on azathioprine maintenance therapy. Currently, lower doses of corticosteroids are used in combination with other immunosuppressive agents or in short courses of high doses to treat acute rejection. Corticosteroids are also used to treat graft-versus-host disease after bone marrow transplantation and to minimize hypersensitivity reactions caused by induction immunosuppressants, such as monoclonal antibodies and antithymocyte globulin.[26]

The major adverse effects of high doses of corticosteroids are myopathy, diabetes, weight gain, fracture, peptic ulcers, gastrointestinal bleeding, opportunistic infections, and poor wound healing.

Antiproliferative Agents

Azathioprine, a purine analogue, has been used clinically since 1963. It changes in the liver to 6 mercaptopurine, then enters the cell to be converted to 6-mercaptopurine ribonucleotide, which resembles inosine monophosphate. This structural resemblance interferes with the cellular synthesis of DNA, RNA, and other cofactors. It acts early during the proliferative cycle of effector T-cell and B-cell clones. Recently, it has been replaced by MMF, which is more effective during the first 1 to 3 years after transplant. The major toxic side effects of azathioprine are bone marrow suppression, hepatotoxicity, and increased risk of malignancy.

The immunosuppressive activity of MMF is through inhibition of the purine synthesis pathway. It is a potent, reversible, noncompetitive inhibitor of inosine monophosphate dehydrogenase. Inosine monophosphate dehydrogenase is an essential enzyme for DNA synthesis in both T cells and B cells; thus MMF selectively blocks proliferation of T cells and suppresses antibody formation by B cells, sparing bone marrow and parenchymal cells, which rely more on the salvage pathway for purine synthesis.[34]

The side effects of MMF include diarrhea, esophagitis, and gastritis. The risk of leukopenia and opportunistic infections is similar in both MMF and azathioprine.[26]

Interleukin-2 Receptor Antagonists

The IL-2 receptor is a complex of several transmembrane polypeptide chains. Daclizumab (Zenapax) and basiliximab (Simulect) are specific monoclonal antibodies that bind to the alpha chain of IL-2 receptors. The clinical use of these agents was associated with no major side effects, such as malignancy or opportunistic infections, when compared to placebo.[35]

Lymphocyte-Depleting Agents

Anti-CD3 antibody (OKT3) is a mouse-derived monoclonal antibody that binds to the CD3 glycoprotein on the T-cell surface, preventing antigen binding to the antigen recognition complex and blocking cell-mediated cytotoxicity. The side effects of OKT3 range from a mild flulike illness to a life-threatening shocklike reaction (cytokine release syndrome), encephalopathy, nephropathy, and hypotension. Cytokine release syndrome can be minimized by high doses of steroids a few hours before administration of OKT3.[36]

Antithymocyte globulin (ATG) is prepared from hyperimmune serum of horses and rabbits that were immunized with human thymic lymphocytes. ATG works by binding to the surface of T cells and depleting both circulating T cells and those within lymphoid organs. Polyclonal ATG causes lymphocyte depletion by complement-dependent lysis, opsonization, and apoptosis, and markedly affects other T-cell receptors by down-regulation or binding.[26] The main side effects of ATG are flushing, fever, anaphylaxis, and serum sickness. Other toxic effects include phlebitis, leukopenia, thrombocytopenia, and nephritis.

Conclusion

It is evident that clinical application of CTA transplants is feasible and remarkably expands the quality of reconstructive options and procedures. However, the ongoing debate is whether it is ethical to commit patients to lifelong immunosuppression for "nonvital" organ reconstructions. The risks and benefits should be carefully weighed for each individual patient before CTA transplantation is warranted. At this point, because the tolerance-inducing strategies are not yet available, the most justified procedures are those in patients who are already on immunosuppressive therapy for the solid organ transplants. The perfect example is the concomitant transplantation of the entire abdominal wall allograft in the recipients of the multivisceral organ transplants.

The technical feasibility and the functional outcomes of CTA transplants are exciting. The introduction of tolerance-inducing strategies will bring CTA transplants closer to the routine armamentarium of reconstructive procedures.

References

1. Lee WP, Yaremchuk MJ, Pan YC, et al. Relative antigenicity of components of a vascularized limb allograft. *Plast Reconstr Surg.* 1991;87:401–411.
2. Gilbert R. Transplant is successful with a cadaver forearm. *Med Trib Med News.* 1964;5.
3. Dubernard JM, Owen E, Herzberg G, et al. Human hand allograft: report on first 6 months. *Lancet* 1999;353:1315–1320.
4. Hettiaratchy S, Randolph MA, Petit F, et al. Composite tissue allotransplantation—a new era in plastic surgery? *Br J Plast Surg.* 2004;57:381–391.
5. Jones JW, Gruber SA, Barker JH, et al. Successful hand transplantation—one-year follow-up. *N Eng J Med.* 2000;343:468–473.
6. Lanzetta M, Petruzzo P, Vitale G, et al. Human hand transplantation: what have we learned? *Transplant Proc.* 2004;36:664–668.
7. Giraux P, Sirigu A, Schneider F, et al. Cortical reorganization in motor cortex after graft of both hands. *Nature Neurosci.* 2001;4:691–692.
8. Petit F, Minns AB, Dubernard JM, et al. Composite tissue allotransplantation and reconstructive surgery: first clinical applications. *Ann Surg.* 2003;237:19–25.
9. Levi DM, Tzakis AG, Kato T, et al. Transplantation of the abdominal wall. *Lancet.* 2003;36:2173–2176.
10. Hofmann GO, Kirschner MH, Wagner FD, et al. Allogeneic vascularized transplantation of human femoral diaphyses and total knee joints first clinical experiences. *Transplant Proc.* 1998;30:2754–2761.
11. Hofmann GO, Kirschner MH. Clinical experience in allogeneic vascularized bone and joint allografting. *Microsurgery.* 2000;20:375–383.
12. Guimberteau JC, Baudet J, Panconi B, et al. Human allotransplant of a digital flexion system vascularized on the ulnar pedicle: a preliminary report and 1-year follow-up of two cases. *Plast Reconstr Surg.* 1992;89:1135–1147.
13. Mackinnon SE, Doolabh VB, Novak CB, et al. Clinical outcome following nerve allograft transplantation. *Plast Reconstr Surg.* 2001;107:1419–1429.
14. Atchabahian A, Mackinnon SE, Hunter DA. Cold preservation of nerve decreases expression of ICAM-1 and class MHC antigens. *J Reconstr Microsurg.* 1999;15:307–311.
15. Evans PJ, Mackinnon SE, Levi AD, et al. Cold preserved nerve allografts: changes in basement membrane, viability, immunogenicity, and regeneration. *Muscle Nerve.*1998;21:1507–1522.
16. Hare GM, Evans PJ, Mackinnon SE, et al. Effect of cold preservation on lymphocyte migration into peripheral nerve allograft antigenicity with warm and cold temperature preservation. *Plast Reconstr Surg.* 1996;97:152–162.
17. Strome M. Human laryngeal transplantation: considerations and implications. *Microsurgery.* 2000;20:372–374.
18. Strome M, Stein J, Esclamado R, et al. Laryngeal transplantation and 40-month follow-up. *N Engl J Med.* 2001;344:1676–1679.
19. Lorenz RR, Hicks DM, Shields RW Jr, et al. Laryngeal nerve function after total laryngeal transplantation. *Otolaryngol Head Neck Surg.* 2004;131:1016–1018.
20. Jones TR, Humphrey PA, Brennan DC. Transplantation of vascularized allogeneic skeletal muscle for scalp reconstruction in a renal transplant patient. *Transplant Proc.* 1998; 30:2746–2753.
21. Birchall M. Tongue transplantation. *Lancet.* 2004;363:1663.
22. Macchiarini P, Lenot B, de Montpreville V, et al. Heterotopic pig model for direct revascularization and venous drainage of tracheal allografts. Paris-Sud University Lung Transplantation Group. *J Thorac Cardiovasc Surg.* 1994;108:1066–1075.
23. Rose KG, Sesterhenn K, Wustrow F. Tracheal allotransplantation in man. *Lancet.* 1979;1(8113):433.
24. Levashov YuN, Yablonsky PK, Cherny SM, et al. One-stage allotransplantation of thoracic segment of the trachea in a patient with idiopathic fibrosing mediastinitis and marked tracheal stenosis. *Eur J Cardiothorac Surg.* 1993;7:383–386.
25. Klepetko W, Marta GM, Wisser W, et al. Heterotopic tracheal transplantation with omentum wrapping in the abdominal position preserves functional and structural integrity of a human tracheal allograft. *J Thorac Cardiovasc Surg.* 2004;127:862–867.
26. Gorantla VS, Barker JH, Jones JW Jr, et al. Immunosuppressive agents in transplantation: mechanisms of action and current anti-rejection strategies. *Microsurgery.* 2000;20:420–429.

27. Liu J, Farmer JD Jr, Lane WS, et al. Calcineurin is a common target of cyclophilin-cyclosporine A and FKBP-FK506 complexes. *Cell.* 1991;66:807–815.

28. Borel JF. Cyclosporine-A—present experimental status. *Transplant Proc.* 1981;13:344–348.

29. Ghasemian SR, Light JA, Currier C, et al. Tacrolimus vs Neoral in renal and renal/pancreas transplantation. *Clin Transplant.* 1999;13(1, pt 2):123–125.

30. Cendales L, Hardy MA. Immunologic considerations in composite tissue transplantation: overview. *Microsurgery.* 2000;20:412–419.

31. Spencer CM, Goa KL, Gillis JC. Tacrolimus. An update of its pharmacology and clinical efficacy in the management of organ transplantation. *Drugs.* 1997;54:925–975.

32. Francois CG, Breidenbach WC, Maldonado C, et al. Hand transplantation: comparisons and observations of the first four clinical cases. *Microsurgery.* 2000;20:360–371.

33. Kahan BD, Podbielski J, Napoli KL, et al. Immunosuppressive effects and safety of a sirolimus/cyclosporine combination regimen for renal transplantation. *Transplantation.* 1998;66:1040–1046.

34. Allison AC, Eugui EM. Immunosuppressive and other effects of mycophenolic acid and an ester prodrug, mycophenolate mofetil. *Immunol Rev.* 1993;136:5–28.

35. Vincenti F, Kirkman R, Light S, et al. Interleukin-2-receptor blockade with daclizumab to prevent acute rejection in renal transplantation. Daclizumab Triple Therapy Study Group. *N Engl J Med.* 1998;338:161–165.

36. Buysmann S, Hack CE, van Diepen FN, et al. Administration of OKT3 as a two-hour infusion attenuates first-dose side effects. *Transplantation.* 1997;64:1620–1623.

3

Advanced Concepts in Vascularized Tissue Transfer in the Hand

Holger Engel and Günter Germann

Introduction

Soft tissue defects in the hand with exposed tendons, bones, or joints often present difficult reconstructive problems.[1-15] These problems are usually related to the limited availability of local flaps and to the technically demanding dissections of their delicate vasculature.[16-24] Microsurgical dissection techniques and a precise knowledge of anatomy are required to successfully release these flaps. Rediscovery of anatomical studies by Spalteholz, Manchot, and Salmon[21,22,25] provided the impetus for modern anatomical studies of the vasculature of the hand.[26-32] These studies in turn led to a new generation of flaps in a wide variety of sizes and from a wide variety of donor sites. Most of these flaps are from the dorso-lateral aspect of the hand and digits; only a few are raised at the palmar aspect.[33-39] In this chapter, we review some advanced concepts of transferring intrinsic flaps of the hand, including complex reconstruction with multiple-component chimeric flaps.

Venous and Arterial Anatomy of the Hand and Fingers

There are two venous systems in the hand: a deep system with small, hardly visible concomitant veins running with the arteries; and a more superficial, large-calibre cutaneous system.[40-43] Venous valves are consistently found in veins with a calibre of 0.2 mm or larger. The only important exception concerning the presence of these valves seems to be the venous arches that allow either radial-ulnar or palmar-dorsal drainage, such as veins close to all joints and subdermal veins on the dorsal, palmar, and lateral surfaces of the hand and fingers. Finally, the orientation of the venous valves indicates that the direction of the venous flow generally is from the palmar to the dorsal side of the hand, and from the superficial to the deep vein system.

All arteries of the hand and fingers originate from the main forearm vessels: the radial, ulnar, and anterior and posterior interosseous arteries. These arteries are the tributaries to the vascularity of the wrist, which appears to be that of two palmar (superficial palmar and deep palmar arch) and three dorsal carpal arches (basal metacarpal arch, dorsal intercarpal arch, dorsal radiocarpal arch; Figures 3-1a and 3-1b).[44-47]

The common digital arteries usually branch off the superficial palmar arch to divide into the radial and ulnar proper digital arteries at the level of the metacarpal head. The palmar metacarpal arteries are fed by the deep palmar arch. After running as a single vessel, each palmar metacarpal artery divides into two and exits laterally from under the palmar plate to cradle the metacarpal head or to connect with a common digital artery. The four dorsal metacarpal arteries are based on the three dorsal carpal arches.[32]

Important for understanding the great versatility of intrinsic flaps based on this network is the fact that each artery connects with the palmar arterial system, both proximally and distally. The main connecting vessel is the palmar perforator in the web space, usually forming the feeding vessel for the dorsal metacarpal artery flap (Figures 3-1a and 3-1b).[32]

Tissue Surgery

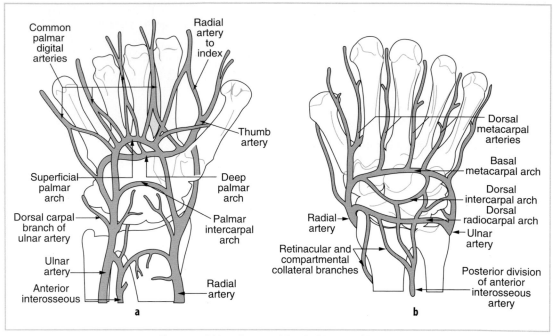

Figure 3-1. (**a**) Arterial anatomy of the palm. (**b**) Dorsum of the hand.

Principles of Intrinsic Flap Design

The rapid evolution of surgical and technical expertise and increasing anatomical and clinical knowledge has lead to a high standard of soft tissue reconstruction of the hand. In contrast to traditional distant pedicle flaps, intrinsic flaps permit immediate wound closure and early active mobilization and physical therapy. This one-stage concept avoids the drawbacks of distant pedicle flaps, such as multiple procedures, extended immobilization, prolonged time off work, and increased treatment cost. Besides a sound knowledge of the anatomy, reconstructing defects in the hand requires an algorithmic approach to select the ideal flap in the particular clinical situation. A thorough analysis of the defect is the first step in the reconstruction algorithm and has to precede the selection of any reconstructive procedure. Decisions are based on the evaluation of 1) the size of the defect, 2) the location of the defect, 3) any missing tissue components, 4) the degree of sensation required, 5) treatment options, 6) contraindications to treatment, and 7) the personal profile of the patient.

All factors need to be assessed to determine whether the defect can be reconstructed by local means or whether a distant pedicle flap, or even a free flap, is indicated. Flap choice also depends more on the patient's profile than on the characteristics of the defect. Whenever possible, the patient's desires and expectations should be discussed before surgery to avoid later problems with unsightly donor sites, impaired mobility of digits, or other possibly unpleasant results.

In addition to algorithmic problem solving, every surgeon has to consider the technical aspects in designing flaps in the hand and fingers. The following principals may appear trivial, but many flap failures can be traced back to an error in planning the flap (Figure 3-2):

1. Adequate flap size;
2. Adequate length and arc of rotation (that is, no tension or kinking of the pedicle);
3. Adequate protection of perfusion (no inappropriate tension on the pedicle flaps);
4. The location of a skin island in an axial island or in dorsal metacarpal flaps; and
5. The location of perforators in axial island flaps.

The quickest, easiest, and safest methods best suited for the patient should be used to obtain the best possible outcome. The ideal solution is considered to be a flap that 1) meets the

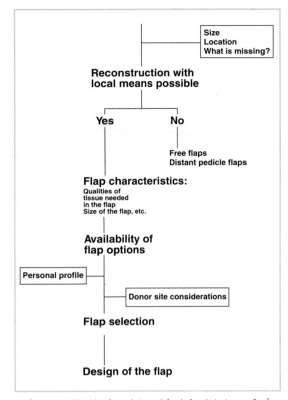

Figure 3-2. Algorithm for analyzing a defect before designing any flap.[2]

requirements of the patient, 2) has acceptable donor-site morbidity, and 3) is the least technically difficult.

Classification of Intrinsic Flaps

Intrinsic flaps, and flaps in general, can be classified according to 1) vascular anatomy, 2) their method of use, 3) the tissue components they include, 4) the perfusion pattern (antegrade or retrograde), or 5) the location of the donor site.

Flaps are generally divided into random-pattern flaps and axial-pattern flaps. Because of the rich vascular network described above, flaps can be based on proximal or distal pedicles. Proximally based flaps are called "antegrade flaps." Flaps that are nourished by distal inflow are called "retrograde flaps."

Traditional Flaps

Several intrinsic flaps have been used in recent decades. Among the more frequently employed are random-pattern flaps, which are the classic cross-finger flap or the thenar flap; and axial-pattern flaps, the prototypes of which were the Littler flap or the Hilgenfeldt flap (later described by Foucher as the "kite flap"), both used as heterodigital flaps for reconstructing the pulp of the thumb. On the basis of these classic descriptions and on additional anatomic studies, modifications, and refinements, new types of flaps have been developed and are described in more detailed below.

Cross-Finger Flaps

The classic "cross-finger" flap has been modified into several forms. All these forms are principally considered to be random-pattern flaps, although small axial cutaneous branches may be included in some modifications, as for example in the C-ring flap, which contains defined vessels to enhance its versatility and mobility.[36] The C-ring flap is either a proximally or distally based flap that consists of the semi-circumference of the digit (Figure 3-3).[48]

The "cross-finger" flap can cover larger complex defects in the distal middle phalanx and can also be re-innervated, but its arc of rotation is limited because of the short pedicle. Therefore, the most important principle in planning a cross-finger flap is to square the defect and to adjust the level of the defect in the digit to the

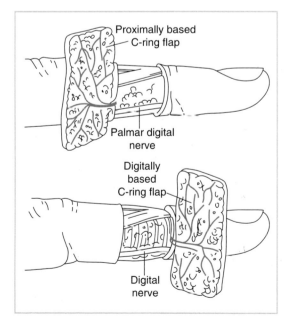

Figure 3-3. Steps in elevating the C-ring digital flap.

level of the flap to avoid tension on the flap. Some temporary flexion of the donor or recipient finger may be necessary to reduce tension on the flap. The largest flap can be raised on the middle phalanx. The paratenon must be preserved to secure grafting at the donor site. Donor site morbidity can be considerable if the semicircumference of the digit is raised.

Reverse Cross-Finger Flaps

Reverse cross-finger flaps are used to repair dorsal finger defects of the adjacent finger.[49] The choice of the donor finger and the donor region is based on the same considerations as in the traditional technique.

The technique follows the "open the door-close the door" principle. After elevating the skin of the donor site as a pedicled vascularized dermal flap ("open the door"), the subcutaneous tissue is elevated in the opposite direction by placing its base adjacent to the recipient finger, preserving the paratenon. The subcutaneous flap is then flipped over like the page of a book and sutured into the defect. After the subcutaneous flap is inset, the pedicled vascularized dermal flap is sewn back into its bed ("close the door"), and a tie-over dressing is applied. A split-thickness skin graft (STSG) is applied to the reversed surface of the reversed subcutaneous flap. Securing the flap with sutures, buddy taping, or k-wire fixation is mandatory (Figure 3-4).

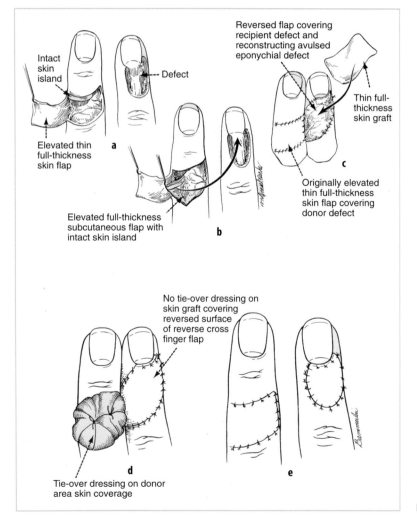

Figure 3-4. Reversed cross-finger flap.[3]

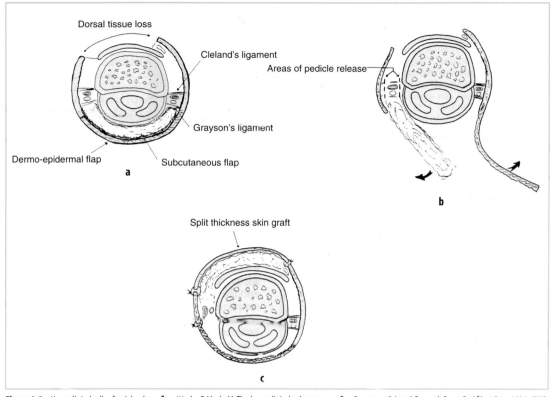

Figure 3-5. Homodigital adipofascial palmar flap. (Voche P, Merle M. The homodigital subcutaneous flap for cover of dorsal finger defects. *Br J Plast Surg.* 1994;47(6): 435–439. Copyright (1994), with permission from The British Association of Plastic Surgeons.)

Variations of Random-Pattern Flaps

Another option to cover a dorsal defect of the finger is a homodigital adipofascial palmar flap, as described by Voche and Merle (Figure 3-5).[31,50] In anatomic studies, they documented the vascular supply of the palmar subcutaneous tissue, and they use this layer as a turnover flap to cover dorsal defects. This flap definitely has potential, but very delicate dissection is required to preserve the paratenon of the flexor tendons and to avoid injuring the neurovascular bundle.

Flaps With Axial-Pattern Perfusion

Axial-pattern flaps are characteristically based on a defined vessel that independently perfuses the area of the flap, either directly or through perforating branches. The design of axial island flaps, most frequently used as digital or dorsal metacarpal flaps, varies substantially from that of a local transposition flap. The size of the flap should match the size of the defect, with only a slight overcorrection. Most surgeons design the skin island slightly larger to avoid any tension on the flap. This is usually tolerated by the flap. Flaps that are too large for the defect may result in venous congestion rather than in additional safety to the flap.

The arc of rotation, which is determined by the length of the pedicle, is of utmost importance for the success of an axial island flap. It is even more important in reverse pedicle flaps. Antegrade flaps usually do not exceed an arc of rotation of 90° to 120°, which greatly reduces the risk of kinking. Reverse pedicle flaps frequently have arcs of rotation of 180°. In these flaps, if the pedicle is not long enough to allow a wide arc, kinking of the pedicle can jeopardise venous outflow. Adding 10% to 15% more length to the pedicle, avoiding the use of narrow tunnels for the pedicle, and using a loose closure of the wound, should be included into the flap design to avoid these complications.

Antegrade and Retrograde Homodigital Artery Flaps

Homodigital island flaps, antegrade or reverse, can be employed to repair various types of defects from complex injuries of the hand, especially when easier techniques, such as cross-finger flaps, are not possible as a result of severe multiple finger injuries.

These flaps rely on one of the digital arteries or on a perforator branching off these vessels, together with their concomitant veins, which are protected on the palmar side by the Grayson ligament and on the dorsal by the Cleland ligament.

A retrograde pedicle is possible by using retrograde blood flow through the finger's palmar arches at the DIP (distal interphalangeal) or PIP (proximal interphalangeal) level,[35,55–57] where a palmar arch runs between the flexor tendon sheath and the bone (Figure 3-6).[58] The integrity of these transverse digital arches is essential for a successful flap. The vascular pedicle is reliable, and the arc of rotation is wide enough to reach the PIP and DIP joints; therefore, these flaps are indicated for distal homo-digital dorsal defects, especially over exposed joints and fingertip injuries, with acceptable donor site morbidity. A full-thickness skin graft for the donor site is required.

Heterodigital Island Flaps

Heterodigital arterialized flaps are useful for resurfacing large defects in the hand, as well as the palmar, dorsal, and lateral aspects of adjacent fingers that are too big for local transposition flaps. The flaps are thin and pliable, and the morbidity to the donor finger is minimal. The flap is based on the digital artery of an adjacent finger, and in some cases includes a vein from the dorsum of the finger. This vein improves flap hemodynamics and prevents venous congestion in the flap, which can occur in island flaps from the fingers that depend solely on the venae comitantes of the digital artery.[59] If a longer reach is required, the heterodigital arterialized flap can be extended by dividing the dorsal vein. Once the flap has been transferred, the venous pedicle of the flap can be reconnected microsurgically.[60] Clinical cases reported by Tai et al. showed complete flap survival with no postoperative venous flap congestion and normal sensation in the donor finger pulp (Figure 3-7).

Heterodigital, Reversed Neurovascular Island Flaps

Heterodigital, reversed neurovascular island flaps are designed on the dorso-lateral aspect of the middle phalanx of the adjacent uninjured finger. They are indicated for repairing extensive defects in fingers that cannot be reconstructed using other flaps and as an alternative to microsurgical reconstruction. The length of the vascular pedicle allows a wide arc of transposition for covering defects in the middle and index fingers. A digital Allen's test and Doppler examination must confirm the patency of the digital arteries of the injured and adjacent donor fingers preoperatively. If a neurovascular flap is to be created, a dorsal sensory branch of the digital nerve can be dissected and attached to the flap.

After dissecting the common digital artery between the injured finger and the flap-donor finger, the artery is transected before its bifurcation; and the digital artery is identified up to its bifurcation in the palm. The converging branches are mobilized as a continuous vascular pedicle for the flap, so that vascularization is provided by a reverse flow through the proximal transverse digital palmar arch of the injured finger.[61] Despite the possibility of one-stage reconstruction, early postoperative mobilization, good functional recovery, and satisfactory cosmetic and sensory results, this technique has disadvantages, which include the sacrifice of the common digital artery, as well as the need to violate a healthy finger.

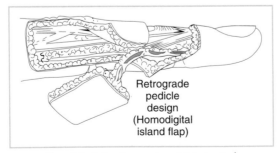

Retrograde
pedicle
design
(Homodigital
island flap)

Figure 3-6. Design of a reverse homodigital artery flap.[1]

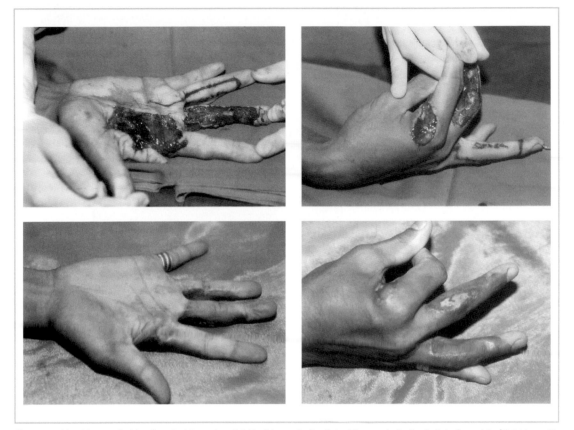

Figure 3-7. (above) Preoperative injury. Extensive injury to the radial side of the palm with damage to the radial digital artery of the index finger precludes harvesting the heterodigital arterialized flap from the ulnar side of the index finger, as this would risk necrosis of the donor finger. As the flap came from the noncontiguous side of the ring finger, vein division was necessary to facilitate transfer of the flap. (below) Postoperative healing. Both the flap and the full-thickness skin graft have healed well. (Tay SC, Teoh LC, Tan SH, et al. Extending the reach of the heterodigital arterialized flap by vein division and repair. *Plast Reconstr Surg.* 2004;114(6):1450–1456.)

Thenar Flaps Based on the Superficial Palmar Branch of the Radial Artery

The classic thenar flap as a random-pattern flap for reconstructing defects of the pulp is well known and has been described by numerous authors.[2,11,14,64–71] In 1993, Kamei et al. introduced the "free thenar flap" based on the superficial palmar branch of the radial artery.[72] This introduction was followed by various vascular and neuro-anatomical studies (Figure 3-8).[11,73–76]

These studies consistently showed that the superficial palmar branch of the radial artery has an average diameter of 1.4 mm and supplies a constant area of skin over the proximal parts of the abductor pollicis brevis and opponens pollicis muscles. After giving off a nutrient branch to the thenar muscle, the superficial palmar artery branch runs through the base of the thenar fascia and consistently gives perforating branches to the thenar fasciocutaneous area. The palmar aspect of the thenar eminence is consistently innervated by the cutaneous branch of the median nerve, and the radial aspect is innervated by the superficial branch of the radial nerve and the lateral antebrachial cutaneous nerve.[11,74,75,77]

Given the anatomy described above, a fasciocutaneous flap can be raised that can also be used as an innervated flap.[75,77] The large diameter of the vessels allows its use as a free flap.[11,72–75,77,78]

In particular defects, such as massive palmar defects and degloving injuries, a flap based on the superficial palmar branch of the radial artery can be combined with a radial forearm flap by extending the vascular pedicle to the radial artery.[77] In about 60% of all people, a distal connection with the superficial palmar arch enables

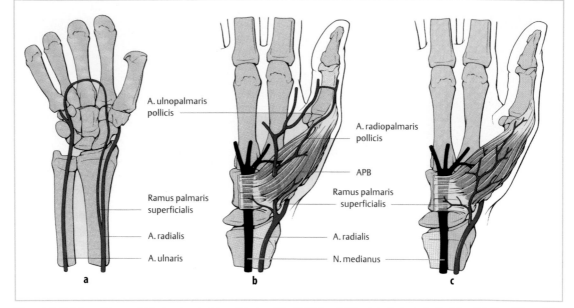

Figure 3-8. Variations of the superficial palmar branch of the radial artery. (Schmidt HM, Lanz U. Chirurgische Anatomie der Hand, New York: Georg Thieme Verlag, 2003.)

the creation of reverse-flow island flaps from the thenar area for reconstructing the thumb or for covering palmar defects after resecting Dupuytren's contracture (Figure 3-9).[11]

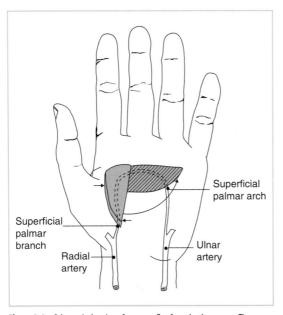

Figure 3-9. Schematic drawing of a reverse flap from the thenar area. The superficial palmar branch of the radial artery connects to the superficial palmar arch, which enables reverse-flow island flaps to cover palmar defects.

Hypothenar Flaps Based on the Ulnar Palmar Digital Artery

The skin over the hypothenar eminence is nourished by musculocutaneous or fasciocutaneous perforator arteries, which pass through the hypothenar muscles or fascia. The distal half of the hypothenar eminence has a constant vascular supply from the ulnar palmar digital artery of the little finger. Innervation of this area is from dorsal or palmar cutaneous branches of the ulnar nerve (Figure 3-10).[10,79–81]

The ulnar hypothenar flap is designed over the ulnar aspect of the distal half of the hypothenar eminence, which is located over the abductor digiti minimi muscle. The flap can include multiple fasciocutaneous perforating vessels that arise from the ulnar palmar digital artery of the little finger.[82–85]

To cover skin and soft tissue defects of the little finger, the flap can be designed and transferred in a retrograde fashion.[82] In these cases, the pivot point is located at the proximal phalangeal level. Sensory innervation of the area is mainly provided by the dorsal branch of the ulnar nerve. In the sensate flap, the innervating nerve is sutured to the palmar digital nerve at the distal phalangeal joint (Figure 3-11).

The arterial blood supply of this reverse flap is ensured by communication between the radial

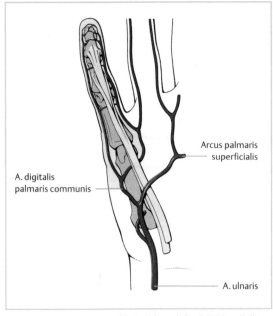

Figure 3-10. Arterial anatomy of the little finger. (Schmidt HM, Lanz U. Chirurgische Anatomie der Hand. New York. Georg Thieme Verlag, 2003.)

and ulnar palmar digital arteries of the little finger, through the dorsal or palmar arterial arcade. Therefore, preoperative digital Allen tests and Doppler examination of the palmar digital arteries are indispensable for assessing the vasculature of the little finger.

In contrast to other conventional flaps , such as the cross-finger flap and the thenar flap, this flap involves a single-stage procedure without prolonged immobilization. It is a versatile flap well suited for complicated finger injuries with substantial palmar tissue defects, and it allows primary donor-site closure without full- or split-thickness skin grafts.

Flaps Based on the Dorsal Metacarpal Network

The dorsum of the hand is increasingly used as a source of various intrinsic flaps, with a wide range of designs and tissue components.[86–88] These flaps are either proximally (antegrade dorsal metacarpal artery) or distally (reverse dorsal metacarpal artery) based.

The distally based flaps in the hand are called "reverse dorsal metacarpal artery flaps" and "extended reverse dorsal metacarpal artery flaps." First detailed in 1990, these flaps are used increasingly.[87,89] More focus on the vascular anatomy in the last decade has clarified the

design, and hence the versatility, of these local flaps (Figure 3-12).[90–93] In 1997, two major developments in the flap were reported:[90] an "extended, reverse, dorsal metacarpal artery flap," designed by Karacalar et al.[92]; and a "reverse dorsal metacarpal artery composite flap" containing a vascular segment of bone. Various authors reported composite flaps including tendon segments.[87,88]

Extended Dorsal Metacarpal Artery Flaps

The extended dorsal metacarpal artery flap is a recently described variation of the dorsal metacarpal artery (DMCA) flap.[94] The arc of rotation can be markedly enlarged by using the first perforator vessel in the proximal phalanx at the most distal base of the flap. This vessel also forms the base of the midphalangeal island flap and feeds the subcutaneous arterial network. The

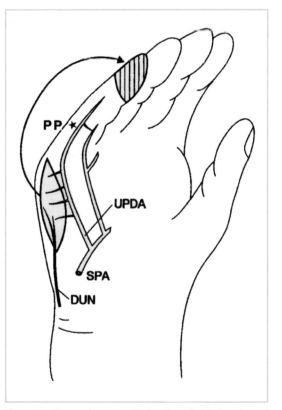

Figure 3-11. Diagram of the reverse ulnar hypothenar flap. The flap is designed over the distal half of the ulnar aspect of the hypothenar eminence. UPDA = ulnar palmar digital artery; PP = pivot point of the reverse flap; SPA = superficial palmar arch; DUN = dorsal branch of the ulnar nerve. (Omokawa S, Yajima H, Inada Y, et al. A reverse ulnar hypothenar flap for finger reconstruction. Plast Reconstr Surg. 2000;106(4):828–833.)

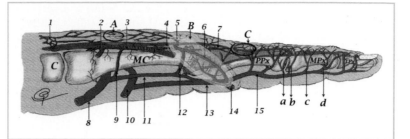

Figure 3-12. Vascular network supplying dorsum of the hand: (1) rete carpi dorsale, (2) dorsal carpal arch, (3) dorsal metacarpal artery (DMCA), (4) junctura tendineae, (5) cutaneous perforator from DMCA, (6) continuation of DMCA to join the confluence of common digital artery and digital arteries, (7) lateral terminal branches of DMCA anastomosing (C) with dorsal branches of digital artery, (8) deep palmar arch, (9) proximal communication perforator between DMCA and palmar metacarpal artery (PMCA), (10) superficial palmar arch, (11) PMCA, (12) distal communicating perforator between DMCA and PMCA, (13) common digital artery, (14) digital artery to the neighboring finger, (15) digital artery to the same finger, (a-d) dorsal branches of the digital artery. (Vuppalapati G, Oberlin C, Balakrishnan G. Distally based dorsal hand flaps: clinical experience, cadaveric studies and an update. *Br J Plast Surg*. 2004;57(7):653–667. Copyright (2004), with permission from The British Association of Plastic Surgeons.)

dorsal metacarpal artery and the interosseous fascia must be incorporated into the pedicle (Figure 3-13).

As in other DMCA flaps, the intertendinous connections have to be divided in some instances and should be repaired after flap transfer. To secure venous outflow, a 1-cm strip of subcutaneous tissue should be included. Flaps based on these distal perforators easily reach the dorsum of the fingertips, nail bed, or the distal lateral aspect of the digits (Figure 3-13).

Composite Dorsal Metacarpal Artery Flaps

The composite, reverse, dorsal metacarpal artery flap is technically more demanding than the conventional dorsal metacarpal artery flap. The segmental blood supply to the metacarpals and extensor tendons[95–97] underlines the importance of including the dorsal metacarpal artery in these flaps. Hence, the dissection must proceed between the extensor tendons, or through one of these tendons when a segment is included in the flap, without disturbing the thin branches of the dorsal metacarpal artery to the bone segment, the tendon segment, and the skin paddle (Figure 3-14).

Vuppalapati et al.[96] used a composite reverse dorsal metacarpal artery flap to bridge a segment of severe comminution of the proximal phalanx with the loss of the segmental extensor tendon in the index finger. This flap included a vascularized segment of extensor tendon from the extensor indicis and cortical bone from the second metacarpal bone. Santa-Comba et al. reconstructed the proximal phalanx of the fifth finger with a compound osteo-fascio-cutaneous dorsal metacarpal flap.[88] Kakinoki et al.[98] treated chronic osteomyelitis in the proximal phalanx of the middle finger by inserting a small piece of the interosseous muscle supplied by a reverse flow of the second dorsal metacarpal artery into the bone marrow space, after radical débridement.

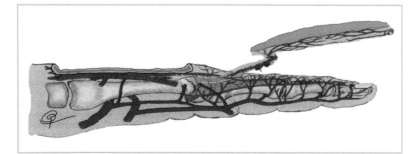

Figure 3-13. Extended reverse dorsal metacarpal artery flap. (Vuppalapati G, Oberlin C, Balakrishnan G. Distally based dorsal hand flaps: clinical experience, cadaveric studies and an update. *Br J Plast Surg*. 2004;57(7):653–667. Copyright (2004), with permission from The British Association of Plastic Surgeons.)

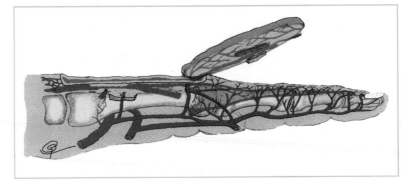

Figure 3-14. Composite reverse dorsal metacarpal artery flap. (Vuppalapati G, Oberlin C, Balakrishnan G. Distally based dorsal hand flaps: clinical experience, cadaveric studies and an update. *Br J Plast Surg*. 2004;57(7):653–667. Copyright (2004), with permission from The British Association of Plastic Surgeons.)

Free "Kite" Flap

The first free microsurgical kite flap was reported by Germann et al. and was developed to reconstruct a residual defect in a replanted thumb.[99] This flap is indicated for reconstructing small defects in the hand for which a pedicled flap is not possible and sensation is needed and as a safe alternative to venous flaps or other free flaps.

The free "kite" flap is a small free flap with thin, stable, and supple skin, providing a long, consistent pedicle with vessels large enough to reconstruct tissue defects outside the area of trauma including a cutaneous nerve that allows restoration of sensation, as in free toe or pulp flaps.

The flap is harvested with the same technique used for the pedicled kite flap from the dorsal aspect of the index finger and includes the first dorsal metacarpal artery, a branch of the superficial radial nerve, and at least one subcutaneous vein.[100,101] Preoperatively, the course of the metacarpal artery must be identified by Doppler sonography. The skin island is outlined on the dorsum of the index finger overlying the proximal phalanx.[102] Wound closure requires skin grafting of the donor defect, ideally with a full-thickness skin graft (Figure 3-15).[100]

Venous Flaps

The so-called venous flaps consist of a variety of flaps based on nutrient perfusion from the venous system. These flaps are used as microvascular flaps to establish arterial perfusion and cannot be considered "intrinsic flaps." Several types Thave been described, either with an antegrade arterial flow through the venous system or as reverse arterialized venous flow-through flaps. They have not yet been widely accepted, but they are favored by a slowly growing number of plastic surgeons.[3,37,103–109]

Vascularized Bone Grafts

The treatment of carpal fracture nonunions or avascular necrosis, such as Kienböck's disease or Preiser's disease, is challenging for the hand surgeon. The goal of surgery is to stabilize and revascularize the affected bone, thereby preventing carpal collapse. These goals can be achieved with vascularized bone grafts and vascular bundle implantations. Numerous authors described different approaches and possibilities for this issue (Figure 3-16).[46,110–137]

The term *therapeutic angiogenesis* describes the induction or stimulation of neovascularization for the treatment or prevention of pathology characterized by local hypovascularity.[138,139] Lunate revascularization is an example of one form of therapeutic intervention, termed *surgical angiogenesis*, which is the surgical transfer of vessels or well vascularized autogenous tissue, alone or augmented with the simultaneous application of vasculogenic cytokines.[140] In hand surgery, both implanted AV bundles and vascularized pedicle or free bone flaps or grafts have been used in the specific case of osteonecrosis.[120,137,140–148] Vascular bundle implantation was established by Hori and Tamai in a canine model.[137] Other authors used lupine and canine autografts,[120,140,149] canine nonvascularized allografts,[141] and dog-to-rabbit nonvascularized

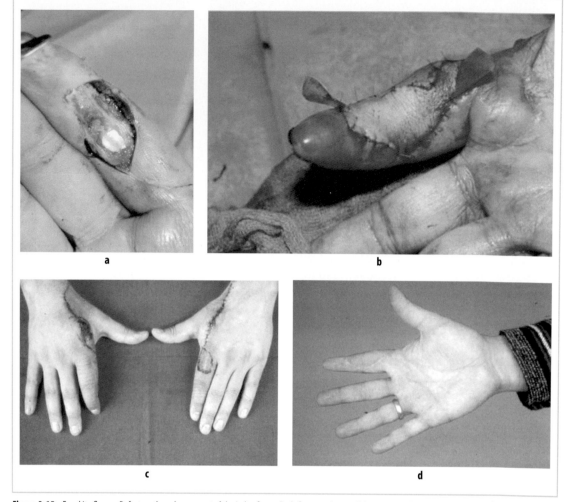

Figure 3-15. Free kite flap. **a.** Defect on the palmar aspect of the index finger. Both flexor tendons and the neurovascular bundles are exposed.[9] **b.** Results intraoperative and **c)** postoperative.[9] **d.** Follow-up 40 months with a good aesthetic result.[9]

xenotransplants.[144] Clinically, this method has been used to treat Kienböck's disease,[147] talar avascular necrosis,[137] scaphoid nonunion with avascular necrosis,[142,145] and in prefabricated-bone free flaps.[143,148,150,151]

Vascularized bone grafts have been described by many investigators and have been transposed from various donor sites, such as the pisiforme bone and the shaft of the radius or ulnar, as well as from the second metacarpal head. Free microvascular transfer of bone from the iliac crest and medial femoral condyle has also been described.[121,124,152–154]

Zaidemberg et al. was one of the first to use reverse pedicled vascularized bone grafts successfully to treat scaphoid nonunion.[132] Mathoulin and Haerle[125] reported a 100% success rate for an antegrade pedicled vascularized transplant from the palmar carpal artery. Technically, the palmar approach is much more challenging than the dorsal because of the proximity of complex anatomical structures. Mathoulin and Brunelli[126] described a technique using pedicled transplantation of the second metacarpal head that had acceptable results. Guimberteau and Panconi[133] employed a bone graft based on

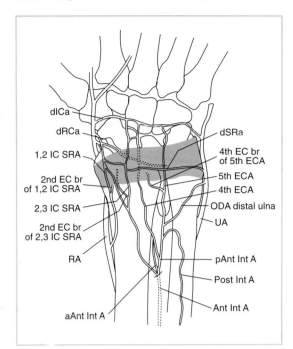

Figure 3-16. Dorsal distal radius and ulna showing extraosseous vessels. aAnt Int A = anterior division of the anterior interosseous artery; Ant Int A = anterior interosseous artery; dICa = dorsal intercarpal arch; dRCa = dorsal radiocarpal arch; dSRa = dorsal supraretinacular arch; 2nd EC br of 1,2 IC SRA = second extensor compartment branch of 1,2 intercompartmental supraretinacular artery; 2nd EC br of 2,3 IC SRA = second extensor compartment of 2,3 intercompartmental artery; 4th EC br of 5th ECA = fourth extensor compartment branch of fifth extensor compartment artery; 4th ECA = fourth extensor compartment artery; 5th ECA = fifth extensor compartment artery; 1,2 IC SRA = 1,2 intercompartmental supraretinacular artery; 2,3 IC SRA = 2,3 intercompartmental supraretinacular artery; ODA, distal ulna = oblique dorsal artery of the distal ulna; pAnt Int A = posterior division of the anterior interosseous artery; Post Int A = posterior interosseous artery; RA = radial artery; UA = ulnar artery.[1]

the ulnar artery with good results. A disadvantage of their technique is the sacrifice of the ulnar artery. Gabl et al.[124] used a free microvascular graft from the iliac crest, but this technique is time-consuming.[114,123] Dai et al.[121] described a bone graft from the supracondylar region of the femur.

Modifications of Vascularized Bone Grafts

Vascularized pedicle bone grafts from the dorsum of the distal radius have been designed on the anatomic studies of Sheetz, Bishop, and Berger.[46,116] Their anatomic studies[46,116] consist-

ently identified several longitudinally oriented vessels that supply nutrient vessels to the dorsum of distal radius.[46] These vessels have consistent spatial relationships to surrounding anatomical landmarks that allow safe dissection and reliable harvest of a segment of vascularized radial metaphysis, which can be transferred as a pedicle graft to the carpus. The radial artery and the posterior division of the anterior interosseous artery are the primary sources of orthograde blood flow to the dorsum of the distal radius (Figure 3-16).

Four vessels that arise from these arteries supply the dorsal radius with nutrient branches. Two are superficial to the extensor retinaculum, providing nutrient branches to the bone underneath the extensor tendon compartments. They are named the 1,2 and 2,3 *intercompartmental supraretinacular* arteries (1,2 and 2,3 IC SRAs). The other two are deep vessels, located on the floor of extensor compartments, named the fourth and fifth *extensor compartmental arteries* (4th and 5th ECAs) for their specific anatomic location in the radial aspect of each compartment. The 1,2 IC SRA courses from the radial artery 5 cm proximal to the radiocarpal joint, beneath the brachioradialis muscle, to emerge on the dorsal surface of the extensor retinaculum. In the anatomic snuffbox, the 1,2 IC SRA anastomoses with the radial artery or the radiocarpal arch (Figure 3-17). This vessel, based on its distal anastomotic connection to the radial artery, is the "ascending irrigating branch" described by Zaidemberg et al.[132] This vessel is actually superficial to the extensor retinaculum, rather than on the periosteum, as originally described.

The 2,3 IC SRA originates from the anterior interosseous artery or the posterior division of the anterior interosseous artery. It is superficial to the extensor retinaculum, directly over Lister's tubercle, and anastomoses with the dorsal intercarpal arch, the dorsal radiocarpal arch, or the 4th ECA. Its nutrient artery branches penetrate deeply into cancellous bone. Like the 1,2 IC SRA, the 2,3 IC SRA can be easily harvested and used as a vascularized pedicle bone graft. The arc of rotation is greater and can reach the entire proximal row, making it useful for either Kienböck's disease or scaphoid nonunions (Figure 3-17).

The 4th ECA originates from the posterior division of the anterior interosseous artery or its fifth extensor compartment branch and

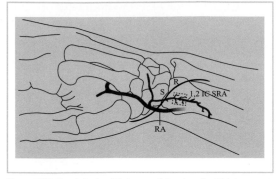

Figure 3-17. Vascularized pedicle bone graft based on the 1,2 intercompartmental supraretinacular artery. The incision is curvilinear, allowing wide exposure for scaphoid vascular bone graft elevation and osteonecrosis visualization.[1]

anastomoses with the dorsal intercarpal and radiocarpal arches. The 5th ECA is the largest of the four dorsal vessels. It is located in the radial floor of the fifth extensor compartment, passing at times through the 4,5 septum. This vessel is supplied by the posterior division of the anterior interosseous artery and anastomoses distally with the dorsal intercarpal arch. Its large diameter, ulnar location (away from required capsulotomy incisions), and multiple anastomoses make it a desirable source of retrograde blood flow. The dorsal radiocarpal arch and the dorsal supraretinacular arch provide important anastomotic connections to these four vessels, allowing each to serve as a distally based or reverse-flow pedicle graft identical in principle to the radial forearm flap. The 1,2 IC SRA was the most useful

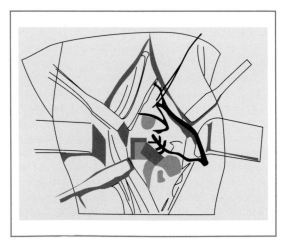

Figure 3-18. Intraoperative view: the 4th extensor compartment artery (ECA) is ligated distal to the bone graft and centered proximal to the radiocarpal joint margin. It is elevated, including the overlying 4th ECA, based on an orthograde 4th ECA pedicle with retrograde flow from the 5th ECA.[1]

for treating scaphoid nonunions and Preiser's disease; and the 5th and 4th ECA was the best pedicle graft for treating Kienböck's disease (Figure 3-18).

To avoid technical pitfalls and to improve clinical outcome, all vascularized pedicle bone grafts must have a pedicle of sufficient length to reach the recipient site without tension. The vascular pedicle should preferably include nutrient vessels that supply both cortical and cancellous bone.[46]

In Kienböck's disease, revascularization with a vascular bundle or vascularized bone graft can be performed even in advanced cases, provided that an intact cartilage shell is present without fracture or fragmentation and no arthrosis is found. Revascularization is a logical alternative to load-altering procedures and is especially attractive in ulnar-neutral or -positive variance cases when radial shortening is contraindicated. Contraindications include stage IV disease and lunate fractures with extrusion or separation of the fragments.

In Preiser's disease, vascularized bone grafts are contraindicated in wrists with level II or III scaphoid nonunion advanced carpal collapse (SNAC) and in wrists with a radiocarpal joint arthrosis.[155] Sauerbier and Bishop[116] reported excellent and promising results with this method that are comparable to the results described above.

The biology and experimental models of fracture healing with vascularized bone grafts have clearly shown the advantages over conventional grafting.[120] Vascularized pedicled bone grafts from the dorsum of the distal radius offer the additional advantage of a single incision for graft harvest and donor site preparation, without potential injury to the palmar carpal ligaments. Faster union times and the ability to revascularize necrotic bone, in addition to the technical ease of harvest, have made these grafts an important tool for hand surgery.

Summary

Intense anatomical studies and resulting modifications of traditional flaps have lead to exciting breakthroughs in the concepts of intrinsic flaps and vascularized tissue transfers in the hand. The variety of options now available has substantially enhanced the reconstructive options, even in complex clinical situations.

References

1. Adani R, Castagnetti C, Landi A. Degloving injuries of the hand and fingers. *Clin Orthop.* 1995;314:19–25.
2. Brown RE, Zook EG, Russell RC. Fingertip reconstruction with flaps and nail bed grafts. *J Hand Surg* [Am] 1999;24(2):345–351.
3. Cheng TJ, Chen HC, Tang YB. Salvage of a devascularized digit with free arterialized venous flap: a case report. *J Trauma.* 1996;40(2):308–310.
4. Germann G, Sauerbier M, Schepler H, et al. Intrinsic flaps in soft tissue reconstruction of the hand. *Perspect Plast Surg.* 1998;11:1–18.
5. Giessler GA, Erdmann D, Germann G. Soft tissue coverage in devastating hand injuries. *Hand Clin.* 2003;19(1):63–71, vi.
6. Hilgenfeldt O. *Operativer Daumenersatz.* Stuttgart: Enke Verlag, 1950.
7. Ishida O, Ikuta Y, Sunagawa T, et al. Abductor digiti minimi musculocutaneous island flap as an opposition transfer: a case report. *J Hand Surg* [Am]. 2003;28(1):130–132.
8. Lister G. Local flaps to the hand. *Hand Clin.* 1985;1(4):621–640.
9. Lister G. *The Hand: Diagnosis and Indications.* 3d ed. Edinburgh: Churchill Livingstone, 1993.
10. Novelino F, Goncalves J, de l'Aulnoit SH, et al. [The fasciocutaneous hypothenar flap: preliminary anatomical and clinical study]. *Ann Chir Plast Esthet.* 2002;47(1):9–11.
11. Omokawa S, Takaoka T, Shigematsu K, et al. Reverse-flow island flap from the thenar area of the hand. *J Reconstr Microsurg.* 2002;18(8):659–664.
12. Rockwell WB, Lister GD. Soft tissue reconstruction. Coverage of hand injuries. *Orthop Clin North Am.* 1993;24(3):411–424.
13. Rose EH. Small flap coverage of hand and digit defects. *Clin Plast Surg.* 1989;16(3):427–442.
14. Takeda A, Fukuda R, Takahashi T, et al. Fingertip reconstruction by nail bed grafting using thenar flap. *Aesthetic Plast Surg.* 2002;26(2):142–145.
15. Vilain R, Dupuis JF. Use of the flag flap for coverage of a small area on a finger or the palm. 20 years experience. *Plast Reconstr Surg.* 1973;51(4):397–401.
16. Adani R, Pancaldi G, Castagnetti C, et al. Neurovascular island flap by the disconnecting-reconnecting technique. *J Hand Surg* [Br]. 1990;15(1):62–65.
17. Eladoumikdachi F, Valkov PL, Thomas J, et al. Anatomy of the intrinsic hand muscles revisited: part I. Interossei. *Plast Reconstr Surg.* 2002;110(5):1211–1224.
18. Eladoumikdachi F, Valkov PL, Thomas J, et al. Anatomy of the intrinsic hand muscles revisited: part II. Lumbricals. *Plast Reconstr Surg.* 2002;110(5):1225–1231.
19. Germann G. Principles of Flap Design for Surgery of the Hand. In: Levin LS, Germann G. *Atlas of Hand Clinics, Local Flap Coverage About the Hand.* Philadelphia: W.B. Saunders, 1998.
20. Goffin D, Brunelli F, Galbiatti A, et al. A new flap based on the distal branches of the radial artery. *Ann Chir Main Memb Super.* 1992;11(3):217–225.
21. Manchot C. Die Hautarterien des Menschlichen Korpers. Leipzig: Verlag von Vogel, 1889. Reprinted in *Rev Arg Cir Plast.* 1991;1:67.
22. Spalteholz W. Die Verteilung der Blutgefässe in der Haut. *Anat Med Phys.* 1893;1:137.
23. Taylor GI, Palmer JH. The vascular territories (angiosomes) of the body: experimental study and clinical applications. *Br J Plast Surg.* 1987;40(2):113–141.
24. Weinzweig N, Starker I, Sharzer LA, et al. Revisitation of the vascular anatomy of the lumbrical and interosseous muscles. *Plast Reconstr Surg.* 1997;99(3):785–790.
25. Salmon M. *Les arteres de la peau.* Paris: Masson Ed, 1936.
26. Bene MD, Petrolati M, Raimondi P, et al. Reverse dorsal digital island flap. *Plast Reconstr Surg.* 1994;93(3):552–557.
27. Earley MJ. The second dorsal metacarpal artery neurovascular island flap. *J Hand Surg* [Br]. 1989;14(4):434–440.
28. Hoflehner H, Pierer G, Steffen J. [Skeletal thumb reconstruction by vascularized metacarpal II transposition. Anatomic study and clinical case reports]. *Handchir Mikrochir Plast Chir.* 1991;23(2):82–89.
29. Hu W, Martin D, Foucher G, et al. [Anterior interosseous flap]. *Ann Chir Plast Esthet.* 1994;39(3):290–300.
30. Sherif MM. First dorsal metacarpal artery flap in hand reconstruction. I. Anatomical study. *J Hand Surg* [Am]. 1994;19(1):26–31.
31. Voche P, Merle M. Vascular supply of the palmar subcutaneous tissue of fingers. *Br J Plast Surg.* 1996;49(5):315–318.
32. Rezende MR, Mattar Junior R, Cho AB, et al. Anatomic study of the dorsal arterial system of the hand. *Rev Hosp Clin Fac Med Sao Paulo.* 2001;59(2):71–76.
33. Inoue T, Ueda K, Kurihara T, et al. A new cutaneous flap: snuff-box flap. *Br J Plast Surg.* 1993;46(3):252–254.
34. Keramidas E, Rodopoulou S, Metaxotos N, et al. Reverse dorsal digital and intercommissural flaps used for digital reconstruction. *Br J Plast Surg.* 2004;57(1):61–65.
35. Kojima T, Tsuchida Y, Hirase Y, et al. Reverse vascular pedicle digital island flap. *Br J Plast Surg.* 1990;43(3):290–295.
36. Mutaf M, Sensoz O, Ustuner ET. A new design of the cross-finger flap: the C ring flap. *Br J Plast Surg.* 1993;46(2):97–104.
37. Nakayama Y, Iino T, Uchida A, et al. Vascularized free nail grafts nourished by arterial inflow from the venous system. *Plast Reconstr Surg.* 1990;85(2):239–245; discussion 46–7.
38. Quaba AA, Davison PM. The distally-based dorsal metacarpal artery flap. *Br J Plast Surg.* 1990;43(1):28–39.
39. Trankle M, Sauerbier M, Heitmann C, et al. Restoration of thumb sensibility with the innervated first dorsal metacarpal artery island flap. *J Hand Surg* [Am]. 2003;28(5):758–766.
40. Nystrom A, Friden J, Lister GD. Deep venous anatomy of the human palm. *Scand J Plast Reconstr Surg Hand Surg.* 1991;25(3):233–239.
41. Nystrom A, Friden J, Lister GD. Superficial venous anatomy of the human palm. *Scand J Plast Reconstr Surg Hand Surg.* 1990;24(2):121–127.
42. Nystrom A, Friden J, Lister GD. Venous anatomy of the thumb and thenar area. *Scand J Plast Reconstr Surg Hand Surg.* 1992;26(2):155–160.
43. Nystrom A, von Drasek-Ascher G, Friden J, et al. The palmar digital venous anatomy. *Scand J Plast Reconstr Surg Hand Surg.* 1990;24(2):113–119.

44. Gelberman RH, Panagis JS, Taleisnik J, et al. The arterial anatomy of the human carpus, part I: the extraosseous vascularity. *J Hand Surg* [Am]. 1983;8(4):367–375.

45. Panagis JS, Gelberman RH, Taleisnik J, et al. The arterial anatomy of the human carpus, part II: the intraosseous vascularity. *J Hand Surg* [Am]. 1983;8(4):375–382.

46. Sheetz KK, Bishop AT, Berger RA. The arterial blood supply of the distal radius and ulna and its potential use in vascularized pedicled bone grafts. *J Hand Surg* [Am]. 1995;20(6):902–914.

47. Berger RA, Weiss A-PC. *Hand Surgery.* Baltimore: Lippincott Williams & Wilkins, 2004.

48. Levin LS, Germann G. *Local Flap Coverage about the Hand.* Philadelphia: W.B. Saunders, 1998.

49. Pakiam AI. The reversed dermis flap. *Br J Plast Surg.* 1978;31(2):131–135.

50. Voche P, Merle M. The homodigital subcutaneous flap for cover of dorsal finger defects. *Br J Plast Surg.* 1994;47(6):435–439.

51. Adani R, Busa R, Castagnetti C, et al. Homodigital neurovascular island flaps with "direct flow" vascularization. *Ann Plast Surg.* 1997;38(1):36–40.

52. Adani R, Busa R, Pancaldi G, et al. Reverse neurovascular homodigital island flap. *Ann Plast Surg.* 1995;35(1):77–82.

53. Niranjan NS, Armstrong JR. A homodigital reverse pedicle island flap in soft tissue reconstruction of the finger and the thumb. *J Hand Surg* [Br]. 1994;19(2):135–141.

54. Yildirim S, Avci G, Akan M, et al. Complications of the reverse homodigital island flap in fingertip reconstruction. *Ann Plast Surg.* 2002;48(6):586–592.

55. Adani R, Marcuzzi A, Busa R, et al. [A reverse vascular autograft finger island flap. A review of 15 cases and of the literature]. *Ann Chir Main Memb Super.* 1995;14(3):169–181.

56. Lai CS, Lin SD, Chou CK, et al. A versatile method for reconstruction of finger defects: reverse digital artery flap. *Br J Plast Surg.* 1992;45(6):443–453.

57. Oberlin C, Sarcy JJ, Alnot JY. [Cutaneous arterial supply of the hand. Application in the creation of island flaps]. *Ann Chir Main.* 1988;7(2):122–125.

58. Zbrodowski A, Gajisin S, Grodecki J. The anatomy of the digitopalmar arches. *J Bone Joint Surg* [Br]. 1981;63-B(1):108–113.

59. Rose EH. Local arterialized island flap coverage of difficult hand defects preserving donor digit sensibility. *Plast Reconstr Surg.* 1983;72(6):848–858.

60. Tay SC, Teoh LC, Tan SH, et al. Extending the reach of the heterodigital arterialized flap by vein division and repair. *Plast Reconstr Surg.* 2004;114(6):1450–1456.

61. Adani R, Busa R, Scagni R, et al. The heterodigital reversed flow neurovascular island flap for fingertip injuries. *J Hand Surg* [Br]. 1999;24(4):431–436.

62. Martin D, Legaillard P, Bakhach J, et al. [Reverse flow YV pedicle extension: a method of doubling the arc of rotation of a flap under certain conditions]. Ann *Chir Plast Esthet.* 1994;39(4):403–414.

63. Legaillard P, Grangier Y, Casoli V, et al. [Boomerang flap. A true single-stage pedicled cross finger flap]. *Ann Chir Plast Esthet.* 1996;41(3):251–258.

64. Dellon AL. The proximal inset thenar flap for fingertip reconstruction. Plast *Reconstr Surg.* 1983;72(5):698–704.

65. Gatewood J. A plastic repair of finger defects without hospitalization. *JAMA.* 1926;87:1479.

66. Fitoussi F, Ghorbani A, Jehanno P, et al. Thenar flap for severe finger tip injuries in children. *J Hand Surg* [Br]. 2004;29(2):108–112.

67. Meals RA, Brody GS. Gatewood and the first thenar pedicle. *Plast Reconstr Surg.* 1984;73(2):315–9.

68. Melone CP, Jr, Beasley RW, Carstens JH, Jr. The thenar flap—An analysis of its use in 150 cases. *J Hand Surg* [Am]. 1982;7(3):291–297.

69. Smith RJ, Albin R. Thenar "H-flap" for fingertip injuries. *J Trauma.* 1976;16(10):778–781.

70. Flatt AE. The thenar flap. *J Bone Joint Surg* [Br]. 1957;39-B(1):80–85.

71. Gatewood. A plastic repair of finger defects without hospitalization. *JAMA.* 1926;(87):1479.

72. Kamei K, Ide Y, Kimura T. A new free thenar flap. *Plast Reconstr Surg.* 1993;92(7):1380–1384.

73. Pilz SM, Valenti PP, Harguindeguy ED. [Free sensory or retrograde pedicled fasciocutaneous thenar flap: anatomic study and clinical application]. *Handchir Mikrochir Plast Chir.* 1997;29(5):243–246.

74. Omokawa S, Ryu J, Tang JB, et al. Vascular and neural anatomy of the thenar area of the hand: its surgical applications. *Plast Reconstr Surg.* 1997;99(1):116–121.

75. Omokawa S, Mizumoto S, Iwai M, et al. Innervated radial thenar flap for sensory reconstruction of fingers. *J Hand Surg* [Am]. 1996;21(3):373–380.

76. Schmidt HM, Lanz U. *Chirurgische Anatomie der Hand.* New York: Thieme Verlag, 2003.

77. Omokawa S, Mizumoto S, Fukui A, et al. Innervated radial thenar flap combined with radial forearm flap transfer for thumb reconstruction. *Plast Reconstr Surg.* 2001;107(1):152–154.

78. Tsai TM, Sabapathy SR, Martin D. Revascularization of a finger with a thenar mini-free flap. *J Hand Surg* [Am]. 1991;16(4):604–606.

79. Zhang FH, Guo YX, Zhong GW. [Anatomical study on reverse flap of dorso ulnar aspect of mid-hand and its clinical application]. *Zhongguo Xiu Fu Chong Jian Wai Ke Za Zhi.* 2002;16(6):395–397.

80. Konig PS, Hage JJ, Bloem JJ, et al. Variations of the ulnar nerve and ulnar artery in Guyon's canal: a cadaveric study. *J Hand Surg* [Am]. 1994;19(4):617–622.

81. Kojima T, Imai T, Endo T. A study on cutaneous vascularity of the hypothenar region and clinical application as the hypothenar island flap. *J Jpn Soc Surg Hand.* 1988;16(3):545–552.

82. Omokawa S, Yajima H, Inada Y, et al. A reverse ulnar hypothenar flap for finger reconstruction. *Plast Reconstr Surg.* 2000;106(4):828–833.

83. Matholuin C, Bahm J, Roukoz S. Pedicled hypothenar fat flap for median nerve coverage in recalcitrant carpal tunnel syndrome. *Hand Surg.* 2000;5(1):33–40.

84. Gu YD, Zhang LY, Zhang GM. Hypothenar flap. *Chin J Hand Surg.* 1992;8(3):865–865.

85. Kinoshita Y, Kojima T, Hirase Y, et al. Subcutaneous pedicle hypothenar island flap. *Ann Plast Surg.* 1991;27(6):519–526.

86. Pelissier P, Casoli V, Bakhach J, et al. Reverse dorsal digital and metacarpal flaps: a review of 27 cases. *Plast Reconstr Surg.* 1999;103(1):159–165.

87. Quaba AA, Davison PM. The distally-based dorsal hand flap. *Br J Plast Surg.* 1990;43(1):28–39.

88. Santa-Comba A, Amarante J, Silva A, et al. Reverse dorsal metacarpal osteocutaneous flap. *Br J Plast Surg.* 1997;50(7):555–558.

89. Maruyama Y. The reverse dorsal metacarpal flap. *Br J Plast Surg.* 1990;43(1):24–27.

90. Dautel G, Merle M. Dorsal metacarpal reverse flaps. Anatomical basis and clinical application. *J Hand Surg [Br].* 1991;16(4):400–405.

91. Dautel G, Merle M. Direct and reverse dorsal metacarpal flaps. *Br J Plast Surg.* 1992;45(2):123–130.

92. Karacalar A, Ozcan M. A new approach to the reverse dorsal metacarpal artery flap. *J Hand Surg [Am].* 1997;22(2):307–310.

93. Pistre V, Pelissier P, Martin D, et al. Vascular blood supply of the dorsal side of the thumb, first web and index finger: anatomical study. *J Hand Surg [Br].* 2001;26(2):98–104.

94. Bakhach J, Demiri E, Conde A, et al. [Dorsal metacarpal flap with an extensive retrograde pedicle: anatomic study and 22 clinical cases]. *Ann Chir Plast Esthet.* 1999;44(2):185–193; discussion 194.

95. Yu GR, Yuan F, Chang SM, et al. Microsurgical second dorsal metacarpal artery cutaneous and tenocutaneous flap for distal finger reconstruction: anatomic study and clinical application. *Microsurgery.* 2005;25(1):30–35.

96. Vuppalapati G, Oberlin C, Balakrishnan G. Distally based dorsal hand flaps: clinical experience, cadaveric studies and an update. *Br J Plast Surg.* 2004;57(7):653–667.

97. Uysal AC, Alagoz MS, Tuccar E, et al. Vascular anatomy of the metacarpal bones and the interosseous muscles. *Ann Plast Surg.* 2003;51(1):63–68.

98. Kakinoki R, Ikeguchi R, Nakamura T. Second dorsal metacarpal artery muscle flap: an adjunct in the treatment of chronic phalangeal osteomyelitis. *J Hand Surg [Am].* 2004;29(1):49–53.

99. Germann G, Raff T, Schepler H, et al. Salvage of an avascular thumb by arteriovenous flow reversal and a microvascular "kite" flap: case report. *J Reconstr Microsurg.* 1997;13(4):291–295.

100. Pelzer M, Sauerbier M, Germann G, et al. Free "kite" flap: a new flap for reconstruction of small hand defects. *J Reconstr Microsurg.* 2004;20(5):367–372.

101. Germann G, Sherman R, Levin LS. *Decision-Making in Reconstructive Surgery: Upper Extremity.* Heidelberg: Springer-Verlag, 2000.

102. Earley MJ. The arterial supply of the thumb, first web and index finger and its surgical application. *J Hand Surg [Br].* 1986;11(2):163–174.

103. Takeuchi M, Sakurai H, Sasaki K, et al. Treatment of finger avulsion injuries with innervated arterialized venous flaps. *Plast Reconstr Surg.* 2000;106(4):881–885.

104. Woo SH, Jeong JH, Seul JH. Resurfacing relatively large skin defects of the hand using arterialized venous flaps. *J Hand Surg [Br].* 1996;21(2):222–229.

105. Fukui A, Inada Y, Maeda M, et al. Venous flap—its classification and clinical applications. *Microsurgery.* 1994;15(8):571–578.

106. Chen CL, Chiu HY, Lee JW, et al. Arterialized tendocutaneous venous flap for dorsal finger reconstruction. *Microsurgery.* 1994;15(12):886–890.

107. Iwasawa M, Furuta S, Noguchi M, et al. Reconstruction of fingertip deformities of the thumb using a venous flap. *Ann Plast Surg.* 1992;28(2):187–189.

108. Fukui A, Inada Y, Maeda M, et al. Pedicled and "flow-through" venous flaps: clinical applications. *J Reconstr Microsurg.* 1989;5(3):235–243.

109. Tsai TM, Matiko JD, Breidenbach W, et al. Venous flaps in digital revascularization and replantation. *J Reconstr Microsurg.* 1987;3(2):113–119.

110. Roux JL. [Vascularized bone transfers in the wrist and hand]. *Chir Main.* 2003;22(4):173–85.

111. Haerle M, Vandeputte G, Mathoulin C. Palmar vascularized bone grafts for scaphoid nonunion. *J Hand Surg [Am].* 2003;28 Suppl 1:56–57.

112. Haerle M, Schaller HE, Mathoulin C. Vascular anatomy of the palmar surfaces of the distal radius and ulna: its relevance to pedicled bone grafts at the distal palmar forearm. *J Hand Surg [Br].* 2003;28(2):131–136.

113. Shin AY, Bishop AT. Pedicled vascularized bone grafts for disorders of the carpus: scaphoid nonunion and Kienbock's disease. *J Am Acad Orthop Surg.* 2002; 10(3):210–216.

114. Gabl M, Lutz M, Reinhart C, et al. Stage 3 Kienbock's disease: reconstruction of the fractured lunate using a free vascularized iliac bone graft and external fixation. *J Hand Surg [Br].* 2002;27(4):369–373.

115. Shin AY, Bishop AT. Vascularized bone grafts for scaphoid nonunions and Kienbock's disease. *Orthop Clin North [Am].* 2001;32(2):263–277, viii.

116. Sauerbier M, Bishop AT. [Possible applications of pedicled vascularized bone transplants of the distal radius]. *Handchir Mikrochir Plast Chir.* 2001;33(6):387–400.

117. Harpf C, Gabl M, Reinhart C, et al. Small free vascularized iliac crest bone grafts in reconstruction of the scaphoid bone: a retrospective study in 60 cases. *Plast Reconstr Surg.* 2001;108(3):664–674.

118. Tu YK, Bishop AT, Kato T, et al. Experimental carpal reverse-flow pedicle vascularized bone grafts. Part II: bone blood flow measurement by radioactive labelled microspheres in a canine model. *J Hand Surg [Am].* 2000;25(1):46–54.

119. Tu YK, Bishop AT, Kato T, et al. Experimental carpal reverse-flow pedicle vascularized bone grafts. Part I: the anatomical basis of vascularized pedicle bone grafts based on the canine distal radius and ulna. *J Hand Surg [Am].* 2000;25(1):34–45.

120. Sunagawa T, Bishop AT, Muramatsu K. Role of conventional and vascularized bone grafts in scaphoid nonunion with avascular necrosis: a canine experimental study. *J Hand Surg [Am].* 2000;25(5):849–859.

121. Doi K, Oda T, Soo-Heong T, et al. Free vascularized bone graft for nonunion of the scaphoid. *J Hand Surg [Am].* 2000;25(3):507–519.

122. Shin AY, Weinstein LP, Bishop AT. Kienbock's disease and gout. *J Hand Surg [Br].* 1999;24(3):363–365.

123. Gabl M, Reinhart C, Pechlaner S, et al. [Proximal scaphoid pseudarthrosis with avascular pol fragment: long-term outcome after reconstruction with microvascular pedicled iliac crest bone graft]. *Handchir Mikrochir Plast Chir.* 1999;31(3):196–199.

124. Gabl M, Reinhart C, Lutz M, et al. Vascularized bone graft from the iliac crest for the treatment of nonunion of the proximal part of the scaphoid with an avascular fragment. *J Bone Joint Surg Am.* 1999;81(10):1414–1428.

125. Mathoulin C, Haerle M. Vascularized bone graft from the palmar carpal artery for treatment of scaphoid nonunion. *J Hand Surg [Br]* 1998;23(3):318–323.

126. Mathoulin C, Brunelli F. Further experience with the index metacarpal vascularized bone graft. *J Hand Surg [Br].* 1998;23(3):311–317.

127. Khan K, Riaz M, Small JO. The use of the second dorsal metacarpal artery for vascularized bone graft. An anatomical study. *J Hand Surg* [Br]. 1998;23(3):308–310.

128. Berger RA, Bishop AT, Bettinger PC. New dorsal capsulotomy for the surgical exposure of the wrist. *Ann Plast Surg*. 1995;35(1):54–59.

129. Bochud RC, Buchler U. Kienbock's disease, early stage 3—height reconstruction and core revascularization of the lunate. *J Hand Surg* [Br]. 1994;19(4):466–478.

130. Pierer G, Steffen J, Hoflehner H. The vascular blood supply of the second metacarpal bone: anatomic basis for a new vascularized bone graft in hand surgery: an anatomical study in cadavers. *Surg Radiol Anat*. 1992;14(2):103–112.

131. Brunelli F, Mathoulin C, Saffar P. [Description of a vascularized bone graft taken from the head of the 2nd metacarpal bone]. *Ann Chir Main Memb Super*. 1992;11(1):40–45.

132. Zaidemberg C, Siebert JW, Angrigiani C. A new vascularized bone graft for scaphoid nonunion. *J Hand Surg* [Am]. 1991;16(3):474–478.

133. Guimberteau JC, Panconi B. Recalcitrant non-union of the scaphoid treated with a vascularized bone graft based on the ulnar artery. *J Bone Joint Surg* [Am]. 1990;72(1):88–97.

134. Martini AK. [Results of vascular pedicled bone transposition in advanced necrosis of the lunate bone]. *Handchir Mikrochir Plast Chir*. 1987;19(6):318–321.

135. Kuhlmann JN, Mimoun M, Boabighi A, et al. Vascularized bone graft pedicled on the volar carpal artery for non-union of the scaphoid. *J Hand Surg* [Br]. 1987;12(2):203–210.

136. Bruser P, Kohler L, Noever G. [Transposition of pedicled pisiform bone in the treatment of stage III lunate malacia]. *Handchir Mikrochir Plast Chir*. 1986;18(5):309–312.

137. Hori Y, Tamai S, Okuda H, et al. Blood vessel transplantation to bone. *J Hand Surg* [Am]. 1979;4(1):23–33.

138. Hockel M, Schlenger K, Doctrow S, et al. Therapeutic angiogenesis. *Arch Surg*. 1993;128(4):423–429.

139. Pevec WC, Hendricks D, Rosenthal MS, et al. Revascularization of an ischemic limb by use of a muscle pedicle flap: a rabbit model. *J Vasc Surg*. 1991;13(3):385–390.

140. Busa R, Adani R, Castagnetti C, et al. Neovascularized bone grafts: experimental investigation. *Microsurgery*. 1999;19(6):289–295.

141. Carneiro R, Malinin T. Vascularized bone allografts: an experimental study in dogs. *J Reconstr Microsurg*. 1991;7(2):101–103.

142. Fernandez DL, Eggli S. Non-union of the scaphoid. Revascularization of the proximal pole with implantation of a vascular bundle and bone-grafting. *J Bone Joint Surg Am*. 1995;77(6):883–893.

143. Hirase Y, Valauri FA, Buncke HJ. Neovascularized bone, muscle, and myo osseous free flaps: an experimental model. *J Reconstr Microsurg*. 1988;4(3): 209–215.

144. Ikebe S, Masumi S, Yano H, et al. Immunosuppressive effect of tacrolimus (FK-506). Bone xenografts in rabbits. *Acta Orthop Scand*. 1996;67(4):389–392.

145. Steinmann SP, Bishop AT. A vascularized bone graft for repair of scaphoid nonunion. *Hand Clin*. 2001;17(4):647–653, ix.

146. Suzuki O, Bishop AT, Sunagawa T, et al. VEGF-promoted surgical angiogenesis in necrotic bone. *Microsurgery*. 2004;24(1):85–91.

147. Tamai S, Yajima H, Ono H. Revascularization procedures in the treatment of Kienbock's disease. *Hand Clin*. 1993;9(3):455–466.

148. Vinzenz KG, Holle J, Wuringer E, et al. Prefabrication of combined scapula flaps for microsurgical reconstruction in oro-maxillofacial defects: a new method. *J Craniomaxillofac Surg*. 1996;24(4):214–223.

149. Suzuki O. Augmented surgical angiogenesis in necrotic bone: correction of avascular necrosis with vascular endothelial growth factor (VEGF). *Microsurgery*. 2004;24(1):85–91.

150. Khouri RK, Upton J, Shaw WW. Prefabrication of composite free flaps through staged microvascular transfer: an experimental and clinical study. *Plast Reconstr Surg*. 1991;87(1):108–115.

151. Khouri RK, Koudsi B, Reddi H. Tissue transformation into bone in vivo. A potential practical application. *JAMA*. 1991;266(14):1953–1955.

152. Doi K, Sakai K. Vascularized periosteal bone graft from the supracondylar region of the femur. *Microsurgery*. 1994;15(5):305–315.

153. Pechlaner S, Beck E. [Reconstructive surgical procedures in scaphoid pseudarthrosis]. *Unfallchirurg*. 1990;93(4):150–156.

154. Pechlaner S, Hussl H, Kunzel KH. [Alternative surgical method in pseudarthroses of the scaphoid bone. Prospective study]. *Handchir Mikrochir Plast Chir*. 1987;19(6):302–305.

155. Sauerbier M, Bickert B, Trankle M, et al. [Surgical treatment possibilities of advanced carpal collapse (SNAC/SLAC wrist)]. *Unfallchirurg*. 2000;103(7): 564–571.

4

Subcutaneous Tissue Function: The Multimicrovacuolar Absorbing Sliding System in Hand and Plastic Surgery

Jean Claude Guimberteau and Joseph Bakhach

Introduction

A still unresolved issue in human physiology is the mechanism of natural organ intermobility. Nevertheless, in front of this physiological phenomenon, incorporating skin, arteries, nerves, tendons, and muscles, we have to ask new questions. But any explanation has to conform with current knowledge and technologies; it cannot rely on observations from the beginning of last century. We mean that our traditional and current universitarian knowledge at the moment is not in conformity with up-to-date observations and has to be revised.

For many decades, we have accepted such terms as elasticity, mobility, hierarchical tissues repartitions, stratifications, and notions of virtual spaces. In reality, when we pinch the skin and tract, we can imagine the complete subcutaneous and skin reshaping in all elements that we move and observe after traction.

Proof of this may be obtained by simply moving one's fingers: during flexion, the flexor tendon moves longitudinally at least 2 cm in the palm of the hand but without any cutaneous translation. For decades, the scientific explanations for this phenomenon were limited to the notion of virtual space or the existence of loose connective tissue, but the biomechanical foundations for these theories were more than vague. In the past 50 years, research has been on the microscopic level; the global concept of mesosphericity has been abandoned. As time has gone by, and as researchers have examined these notions more closely, new hypotheses have emerged concerning the organization of the subcutaneous tissues.[1,2,3]

Microanatomical Observations In Vivo

We have performed 95 video observations with functional analyses, either directly under the skin or close to tendons, muscle, or nerves sheaths, during surgical human dissections, using light microscopy (magnification ×25).

This gliding or sliding of tissue, which is traditionally called "connective" or "areolar" or "loose tissue and paratenon around the tendons," has been for a long time considered to be "packing tissue," which fills spaces between and within organs. In reality, this tissue has a mechanical finality, allowing movements between the structures it connects, preserving mobility and independence between organs and, in particular, between tendons and skin. This tissue is important to the nutrition of the structures embedded in it and as a frame for blood and lymph vessels.

Its mechanical importance is major; it diminishes friction while allowing easy deformability. Composed of intertwining multidirectional filaments, which create partitions enclosing vacuolar shapes, this tissue is called the multimicrovacuolar collagenous absorbing system (MVCAS) to emphasize its functional impact (Figure 4-1).

This tissue has been studied very little because it had been explained in previous decades by the concept of virtual space or of different fascia repartition with stratification into superficial or profound layers.

Given new information from dissections of fresh or formalin-treated cadavers, the time has come to confirm some anatomical truths about this tissue and to definitively discard certain preconceived ideas.[4]

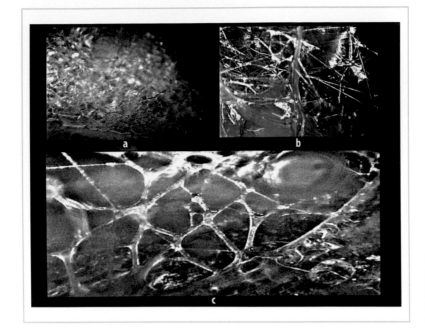

Figure 4-1. a) Traction on the paratendon during surgery. **b)** Searching for an epitendinous plane. **c)** Network between the tendon and the peripheral system: the MVCAS. (A.D.F. Video-Productions with special permission)

Traditional concepts are at variance with anatomical reality. The notion of multilayered sliding between completely anatomically separated tissues—sliding thanks to a so-called elasticity process—has to be revised in light of all these observations. For us, there are no superficial or profound fascia; this distinction is obsolete.

"Microvacuola" and the Microvacuolar Collagenic-Absorbing System

We studied human and animal tissue samples, such as the flexor carpi radialis in cattle, in which the organization of the collagenous system is similar to that of the human flexor profundus muscle.

The sample was prepared by treating it with potassium bichromate, then formalin, and finally caustic soda, thus allowing for softer and more complete hydrolysis. The sample was then frozen and freeze-dried under standard conditions for dehydration. Afterward, it was dissected under binocular magnification. Samples were taken, given a gold-metallic finish, and observed under an electron microscope.

This collagenous system, traditionally called the "paratendon," surrounds the tendon. It is composed of multidirectional filaments, intertwining and creating partitions that enclose vacuolar shapes. This system is called the multimicrovacuolar collagenous absorbing system (MVCAS), to emphasize its functional implication.

This system is situated between the tendon and its neighboring tissue and seems to favor optimal sliding. The tendon may go far and fast without any hindrance and without provoking any movement in neighboring tissue, thus accounting for the absence of any dynamic repercussions of such movement on the skin surface. The movement of the flexor tendon is barely discernible in the palm. It is also the same under the skin areolar tissue, which is the connective link between muscle, tendon, fat aponeurosis, and subdermal areas.

Electron scanning microscopy demolished the theory that the collagenous system consisted of different superimposed layers—layers that were never observed. Furthermore, the elementary laws of mechanics and rheology presented the problem in terms of global dynamics, with the necessity for continuous matter, made up of millions of vacuoles, each one measuring from a few microns to a few millimeters or more, organized in a dispersed branching pattern. We want to express that the living matter is built of microvacuoles.

Microvacuola

The vacuoles measure from a few microns to a few millimeters or more in size and are organized in a dispersed branching fractal pattern.[5] Most of these sequences have a pseudogeometric shape of a polygon. However, they are organized differently according to their function.

All of the vacuoles are situated within a pseudopolygonal fibrillar framework containing a gel. The major role of this framework is to make sure that when stimulated, the structures can move freely without anything else moving around them. The vacuolar structure must be resistant, adapt to the physical forces applied to it, and keep its shape. In other words, its role is to ensure the dynamics of movement and to resist the shocks that this movement creates. The structure also has a memory so that it returns to its initial position between movements (Figure 4-2).

The sides of the vacuoles, which are intertwined, are composed of collagen fibers, mostly type I (23%), III, IV, and VI. They are organized on several levels in different directions, but have no regular, basic pattern. Their diameter ranges from a few to several dozen micrometers, and they vary in length, thus giving an overall disorganized, chaotic appearance. Magnification reveals lateral modifications of the collagen fibers in the vacuole, suggesting the linking of proteoglycan chains. These vacuoles contain a highly hydrated proteoglycan gel (70%) that can change shape during movement but whose volume remains constant. Their lipid content (4%) is high.

Proteoglycans are proteins that are glycosylated by covalent attachment of highly anionic glycosaminoglycans (sulfated polysaccharides). As a result of their strong negative charge, glycosaminoglycans attract counter-ions and water molecules into the tissue. This ability endows proteoglycans with their unique physical characteristics, allowing them to fill the intravacuolar spaces and to change shape when required.

The bonds between the collagen fibrils and the proteoglycan-enriched vacuolar fluid might be composed of type VI collagen, a unique collagen that occurs in the form of beaded filaments and that is often found at the interface between type I collagen and the surrounding extracellular matrix. Type VI collagen is composed of both globular domains and a short, triple-helical domain (60 nm long), and it assembles to form a structure resembling a pearl necklace. Collagen I fibrils also interact specifically with small proteoglycans, such as decorin, whereas large proteoglycans provide hydration and swelling

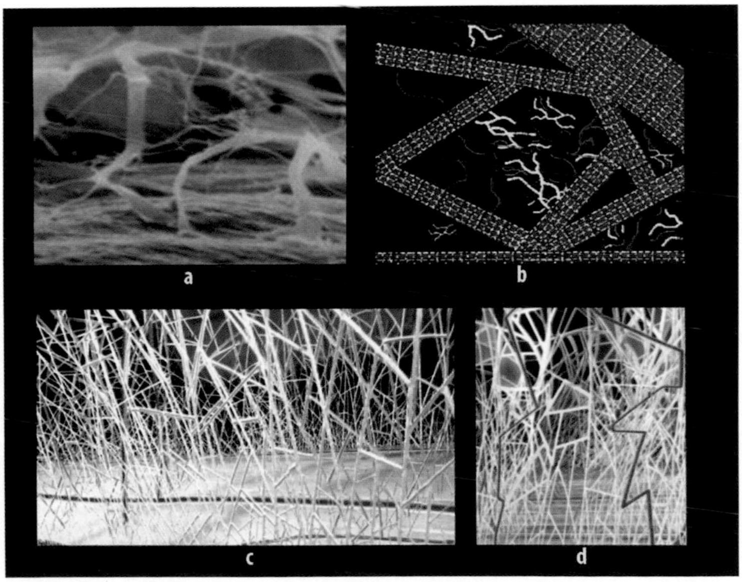

Figure 4-2. MVCAS under the electron microscope. **a)** Histological and collagenous continuity between the epitendon and MVCAS. **b)** Sketch of this organization, in vacuoles. **c)** 3D tissue supports. **d)** 3D vacuola. (A.D.F. Video-Productions with special permission)

pressure, often in association with the nonsulfated glycosaminoglycan hyaluronan. Owing to their capacity to attract water molecules, large proteoglycan molecules allow MVCAS to resist compression, unlike collagen fibrils, which resist tension by extending and retracting under mechanical stress. The collagen framework and the intravacuolar spaces give form and stability to the tissue.

Microvacuola Biomechanical Behavior: A Dynamic Absorbing System

Tissue adaptation to mechanical stress would seem to have two aspects: 1) ensuring the complete movement of the tendon and 2) preserving peripheral tissue stability. How does the MVCAS accomplish these tasks?

The system of microvacuolar networks, in spite of its chaotic aspect, works according to a certain number of rules.[6]

A Chaotic Pattern Dynamic System

The fibrillar framework of the vacuoles is pseudogeometric, polygonal, and tends to be similar to pseudoicosahedral so that it can modify its shape and fill space as it occupies surfaces as efficiently as possible. Although the global aspect of the structure is chaotic, the hierarchically arranged, fractally shaped vacuoles form large pseudopolyedral framework, which may span several partial subunits, and even shift back and forth. The resulting configuration is highly efficient, combining great mechanical strength and lightness. This flexible, pre-stressed polygonal architecture is able to assume many shapes, thereby providing stability and sliding, leading to better metabolism and therefore prolonging the life of the tissue. This tendency to geometric forms is intriguing because it is found in all levels of living matter and seems to be the building block that has developed during the course of evolution.

If the microvacuolar system is thought of as a shock absorber, the resistance it offers is first minimal and then increases as the load increases. Nevertheless, as a shock absorber, its function is to maintain the peripheral structures close to, but not in contact with, the bodily action in progress. The rheological relationship; that is, the local relationship between restraint and distension, cannot be an unlimited, linear, and elastic system, nor can it behave plastically with a limiting plateau. On the contrary, it behaves more like rubber because the collagen fibers cannot be stretched indefinitely but may suddenly rupture. Therefore, why the vacuoles closest to the moving structure undergo maximal deformation whereas those the farthest away hardly change shape is a question that remains to be answered (Figure 4-3).

The fibers rearrange themselves in response to the local stress, thereby explaining the so-called final linear stiffening resulting from the application of the stress: as the stress increases, the fibers become more aligned in the direction of the stress. However, the energy stored in the fibers under tension gradually becomes lower the greater the distance from the stress, so the forces resulting from the pseudolinear stiffening are absorbed, and the structures become stabilized.

We refer to this notion as "combined transmitted and absorbed stress"; that is, each fiber is prestressed and connected to its neighboring fiber by a molecular adhesive link. When tension is applied to the link, the adjacent element undergoes tension and decreases in size little by little until it deforms. All of the component parts then turn so as to be oriented as far as possible in the direction of the applied force, which is controlled to avoid rupture. This interplay between vacuoles and fibrils creates mechanical stability between the forces of local compression and overall tension. The resulting equation is one of equilibrium, maintaining shape, and transmission of information.

Thanks to these explanations, it is easier to understand how the sliding system between many tendons inside the common carpal sheath provides complete independence between the tendons of each finger.

MVCAS and Globality

This sliding tissue is totally continuous throughout the fibers and their prolongation. Even the intermediary structures, such as the deep premuscular fascia, are incorporated in this network and are connected with it on their superior and inferior faces, thereby increasing the shock-absorbing properties of the tissue and allowing the structures to move interdependently. Whether

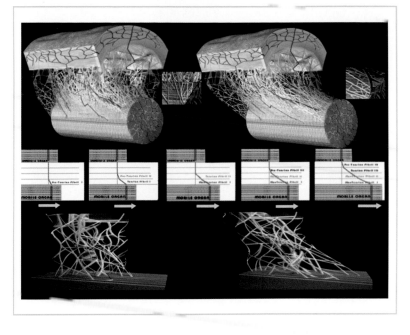

Figure 4-3. Notion as "combined transmitted and absorbed stress." Tension is applied to the link, the adjacent element undergoes tension and decreases in size little by little until deformation occurs. All of the component parts then turn so as to be oriented as far as possible in the direction of the applied force. (A.D.F. Video-Productions with special permission)

it is in the abdominal, thoracic, dorsal, antebrachial regions, or in the scalp, this tissue network is omnipresent. Indeed, there is no space or wall where it is not to be found. Even structures subject to little movement, such as nerves and the periosteum, are surrounded by this fibrillar tissue network, but with differences in the network itself and in the size of the vacuoles.

Indeed, it seems that MVCAS occurs everywhere in the body and that it allows structures to adapt either to internal constraints or to the external environment. Seen in these terms, the whole structure of the body may be considered as an immense collagen network, differing according to the roles it must perform and the stresses it must undergo. In fact, MVCAS and the human body would seem to be one and the same tissue. Living matter has developed within the framework of a multimicrovacuolar chaotic system, including every cell[8] and has acquired a form thanks to physical forces[9] which have subjected it to an increasing complexity within time and space.

MVCAS After Trauma or Pathology

This sliding tissue is supposed to evolve, and each time there is a change in the mechanical constraint (pressure, weight, temperature, ageing),

there is a physiological response and adaptation to the new mechanical situation.

The MVCAS is a very fragile tissue that is based on a precise balance between the frame, composed of collagen molecules, and the inside of the vacuola of glycolicans under pressure.

However, as the mechanical stresses change, as the pathologies appear and unforeseeable need arises to adapt, others factors such as inflammation, edema, aging, trauma, obesity intervene to create changes in shape (Figure 4-4).

Edema is the simplest state of aggression. It can be accommodated with intravacuolar hyperpressure and collagenic distension and without any organic tissue destruction. But the fibrillar distraction caused by intravacuolar hyperpressure is then unable to distend further, and as a consequence, to insure movement. Generally, restitution ad integrum will be the rule.

Open trauma completely destroys the MVCAS harmony and balance. Hemorrhage, liquid extravasations, edema, and hypermia will disturb the mechanical balance, and the sliding system will demand more strength against resistance. Movement will be difficult. Therefore, tissues will become adherent, which will perturb mobility.

This disruption is also the case during inflammation, such as in tenosynovitis or tendinitis. Hypermia, vasodilatation, and local temperature

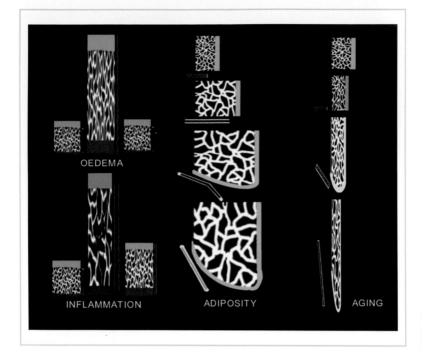

Figure 4-4. MVCAS and physiopathologies. (A.D.F. Video-Productions with special permission)

increases induce intravacuolar hyperpressure with fibrillar dilaceration, creating small megavacuola and completely perturbing movement. Therefore, tissue is destroyed, and the restitution ad integrum will never be obtained. Functional sequelae will be the consequence.

Aging is a very different mechanism. It is not sudden change but rather slow and progressive change in the physical balance of forces inside human tissue. Ageing, because of the loss of internal basic qualities of the MCVAS, is the manifestation of the gravitational "revenge" on the MVCAS internal pre-tension.

This is not the case for obesity, which can be a casual circumstance. It is easy to understand that the vacuola is filled by adipocytes replacing glycolicans. At the beginning, vacuola and fibers are in distension, movement is slowed, and gravitation becomes more important. But this first stage is reversible, thanks to a progressive loss of weight, which must not be too quick.

In the second stage, weight is increasing, and vacuola are in extreme dilatation. Then, fibers are not only in distension but because of the effects of gravitation, they are in dilaceration and in search of a megavacuola transformation, which in turn will be filled by adipocytes. So, body form changes with obesity. At this stage, a return to the original morphology is impossible,

and only surgery will recreate tissue tension by resecting excess skin and fat.

Anatomical Conclusions

This new concept of MVCAS enables us to discuss some basic and traditional assumptions about the nature of tissue and, particularly in hand anatomy, to discuss physiology and reconstructive surgery.

Some traditionally held concepts are at variance with anatomical reality and should be changed. The time has come to confirm some anatomical truths and to discard definitively certain preconceived ideas about the hand. For example, the time-honoured layout of the sheaths in the hand must be completely reconsidered. The notion of a histological difference between the paratendon and the carpal sheath, and the traditionally accepted notion of a piston machine mechanism for sliding phenomenon must also be reconsidered.

When this pressure increases, the balance is disturbed, and the system response is a change in a big vacuola with destruction or local distension of this collagenic frame, which is unable to resist the pressure. When this hyperpressure is caused by an internal situation, such as a ligament (but also by repetitive external movements), the fibrillar framing ruptures, dilates, and then becomes diluted. All of these zones with bigger vacuolar organizations then join many others, forming a megavacuola with cell metaplasia at the inner surface, new biomechanical response more adapted for preserving lubrification, gliding, and adapted volumes. This transformation can be observed all along the flexor or extensor tendon sheaths.

We can find 4 basic types of MVCAS transformations (Figure 4-5):

1. Type I is the basic sliding system surrounding all the tendons, without any external mechanical stress.
2. Type II shows a megavacuola involving, but blood supply is still preserved in protected areas.
3. Type III is under strong constraints with a big megavacuola, and only a few zones for blood supply, thanks to vincula.
4. Type IV has no external blood supply.

This transformation can be also observed during a human's life. At the posterior face of the elbow (the olecranon), hygroma can be noticed, and hygroma is a transformation of the MVCAS organization caused by daily repetitive external pressure all life long.

This transformation can also be observed when draining large collections of subabdominal lymphoceles a few weeks after parieto-abdominal hematoma. The big cavity that results is a megavacuola with inner metaplasia.

Contrary to previous reports, the extension of the digital vascular system is not less effective. It adapts itself in a very different manner, so that vascular flow persists. This is particularly the case in the digital canal, where the hypothesis that the tendon is less well vascularized and fragile is incorrect. The method of functioning is simply different as a result of circumstances in the digital canal, where tendon traction produces articular flexion. The relationship between tendon movement and the resulting digital morphology is geometric—almost linear—and is very different from the situation that pertains in the palm.

Furthermore, this digital movement creates sudden high pressure with anterior compression zones that are incompatible with a vascular epitendineum system. If the palmar system were to exist in the digit, it would lead to intrasynovial bleeding. Therefore, the vessels must be dorsally positioned, the supply network being limited to the protected zones that are near the articular zones and can therefore accommodate tendon excursion, avoiding the stricture and compression that would occur if the vessels were anteriorly placed, just deep to the joint flexion fold.

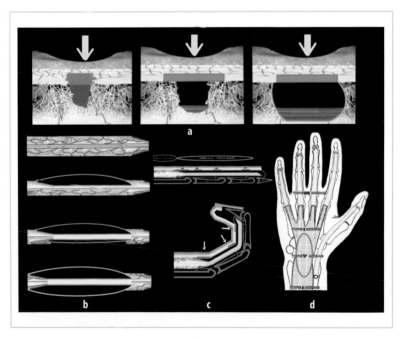

Figure 4-5. a) The MVCAS disappears in its basic network under mechanical constraint and adapts to the new situation with a megavacuola response. **b)** Different MVCAS distributions in the common carpal sheath. **c)** The digital canal is an efficient adaptation of the MVCAS as a megavacuola with vincula: type III. **d)** A proposed new layout of the sliding sheaths in the finger flexor system. (A.D.F. Video-Productions with special permission)

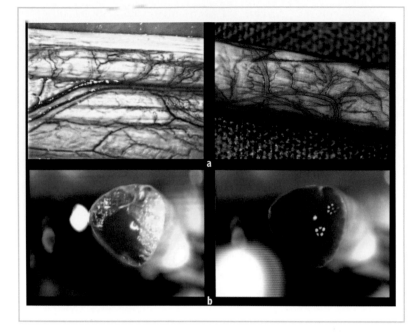

Figure 4-6. Vascularization is continuous and permanent. **a**) Tendons are not hypovascular. Like every organ, vascularization is adapted to its function. **b**) Bleeding of the flexor profundus at A3 pulley level. (A.D.F. Video-Productions with special permission)

There are three joints and three vincula. In fact in Latin, it would be *vinculae*. The vascular anatomy ensures the digital tendinous blood supply under extreme biomechanical stress. The supply is comparable to a skin structure, and our computerized studies repeatedly challenge the hypotheses that propose less well vascularized zones in the flexor tendon. Tendon and epitenon vascularizations are continuous.

The notion of tendon hypovascularization is popular, but its popularity is waning, and to continue to believe in it compromises our vision of tendinous vascularity.

The true situation can be verified by looking at the sequential pictures of tendon vascularization in zones III, IV, and V, showing real blood flow (Figure 4-6).

Like every organ, the vascularization of the tendon has adapted to its function. The notion of the nature of mechanical function between the digital sheath and the carpal sheath and the notion of the preputial string also have to be deeply discussed.

Vascularization is continuous and permanent. There is no area without blood supply. Tendon, epitenon, and MVCAS are supplied by the same vascular system. Tendons are not hypovascular. All of these observations are innovative, in that they introduce a new concept: the sliding unit composed of the tendon and its surrounding sheaths.

Our foregoing observations, which are evidence of real histological continuity between the paratenon, the common carpal sheath, and the flexor tendons, show the perfect vascularization of this functional ensemble.

From now on, any inclination to accept Potenza's principle, tendon adhesions, and reconstruction of the digital sheath using a silicon rod should give way to other principles:

• A tendon has optimal function only when it is surrounded by its original sliding sheath and its vascular heritage.

• A tendon only adheres when it is artificially separated from its own sliding sheath or when the harmony between the tendon and the sheath has been interrupted.

• A tendon is only one of the intervening elements in the transmission of a force through the sliding unit.

For zones III, IV, and V, we wanted to define a different role for the tendon, in the realization and the transmission of a force. The tendon is not a transmission belt acting in the carpal sheath surrounded by a virtual space; nor is it an organ that is avascular or only very slightly vascularized. The tendon is not nourished by the synovial fluid but by its own vascular system, like every organ. The tendon is one of the main constituent elements, but it can no longer be dis-associated from its sheath, thanks to MVCAS.

Physiological Conclusions

There is no histological difference between the paratendon and the carpal sheath. The ancient term *paratendon* thus includes the whole of the peripheric sliding system called multimicrovacuolar collagenic absorbing system, which is made of billions of microvacuolas and fibers frame. The MVCAS is the proximal histological continuation of the perimysium profundus layer, and it differentiates functionally to become the digital sheath. In fact, it is the same structure seen from different aspects under different mechanical circumstances. As soon as an external or internal factor increases internal pressure, the distribution changes in a megavacuola, with a selective blood pedicle in protected areas.

The notion of a piston machine mechanism is false and obsolete and must be replaced by a systemic concept. There is not a duality between the vascular system in the tendons and a peripheral synovial vascular system without communication.

The digital canal is an efficient adaptation of the MVCAS as a megavacuola with vincula system. So the digital and carpal sheaths do not have the same sliding system.

Surgical Conclusions

Vascularized Flexor Tendon Island Forearm Transfer. This new manner of understanding the tendon physiology introduces a completely different concept of reconstruction:

- It emphasizes the tendon-sheath couple and the major role of tendon vascularization with peripheral collagen organization.
- It is inspired by biological consequences and proposes the transfer of a sliding unit composed of a flexor tendon and its surrounding sheaths in a reverse-island-pedicle manner in one single operation, thus avoiding the two-stage procedure for secondary repair (Figure 4-7).

This new technique is used today in clinical cases to reconstruct finger flexor systems in grades III and IV of Boyes's classification.

Two basic principles of this new concept have to be respected. That is, the tendon can only be conceived of 1) as vascularized, and 2) as an element in association with its surrounding sheaths to form a sliding unit.

To conform to these two basic principles, the proposed new technique must satisfactorily answer three basic questions:

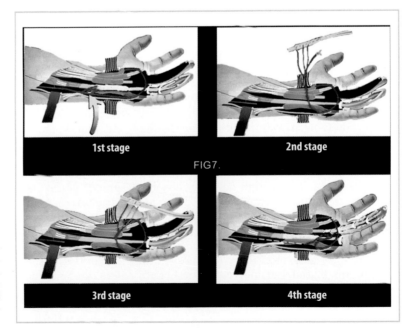

Figure 4-7. The transfer of a sliding flexion unit composed of a flexor tendon and its surrounding sheaths in a reverse island pedicled manner. 1st stage: Mesotendon identification. 2nd stage: Section of FSIVth flexor sublimis of the ring finger and ulnar pedicle. Island ulnar tendon transfer isolated. 3rd stage: Insertion of the island transfer into digital zone. 4th stage: Tendon sutures outside of the No Man's Land and pulley reconstruction. (A.D.F. Video-Productions with special permission)

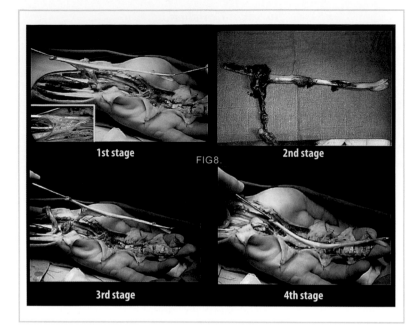

1st stage   FIG8.   2nd stage

3rd stage   4th stage

Figure 4-8. 1st stage: The mesotendon and ulnar artery branches. Flexor superficialis section at the tendinomuscular junction and at the level of decussation. 2nd stage: The flexion sliding unit after revascularization. 3rd stage: Forward translation of the sliding unit transfer. 4th stage: Before inserting and pulley reconstruction. (A.D.F. Video-Productions with special permission)

1. Which sliding zone must be used to replace zones I and II, subject to so many problems and complications?

The mesotenon and its vascular branches provide real vascularization of the flexor tendon and the sliding carpal sheath, both extrinsically and intrinsically. The structure thus transferred is a real sliding structure that already exists in a natural state in zones III, IV, and V.

The principle is to replace the digital sliding zones I and II, the most frequently reconstructed zones, by the natural sliding zones of the wrist and the palm, that is, zones III, IV, and V. Because the tendon used for the reconstruction is transferred with its own sheath, it does not need adhesion with the neighboring tissue to survive, and any adhesion formation is reduced, leading to improved functional results.

Potenza's basic principle of the absolute necessity for adhesion can thus be discarded. The two-stage procedure is now considered obsolete. Furthermore, the transferred tendon is a real flexor tendon with all its original qualities of resistance and flexibility. Technically, the sutures are placed outside "No Man's Land," and the sliding unit, composed of the tendon and the carpal sheath, is inserted between pulleys A1 and A4.

2. What will be the vascularization of the replacement flexion structure? Vascularization is ensured by a preretinacular mesotenon, with branches issuing from the ulnar artery (Figure 4-8).

Anatomical reminder: at the inferior third of the wrist, just before the flexor retinaculum carpi or the annular ligament, the ulnar artery gives off two or three branches about 1 mm in diameter. These branches pass through the common carpal sheath toward the superficial flexor tendons, especially those of the middle finger, the ring finger, and the little finger, by way of a fine transparent mesotenon, which acts as a mesentery. This vascular approach to the flexor system and the common carpal sheath is made distal to the tendon-muscle junction, thus permitting the adaptation of the concept of retrograde island transfers to purely tendinous structures.

This vascularization is one of the principal differences from the radial artery-based flap because it is developed in the tendon zone and not in the muscle zone. Purely tendinous transfers can be founded on the concept of vascularized tendon island transfers, which represents a fundamental change in the concept of tendon reconstruction.

According to the same principle, and using the same surgical technique, it is possible to carry out not only pure tendinous vascular transfers (most often with the superficial flexor tendon of the ring finger), but also a cutaneo-tendinous transfer, and even the triple transfer of skin, tendon, and bone.

3. How will this sliding unit be placed into "No Man's Land"?

Nowadays, the technique of island retrograde forearm transfer is used to transfer a forearm or wrist structure that is pedicled on an arterial axis. For retrograde vascularized tendon transfer, only the ulnar-based pedicle is suitable, owing to its distally based palmar point of rotation and to its branch transmission at an exclusively tendinous level.

Combined Flexor Tendon and Skin Island Forearm Transfer. In some cases, when the overlying skin is extremely scarred and of poor quality, particularly at the base of proximal or middle phalanx, it is impossible to replace the flexor tendon and achieve early motion. Skin of this sort inevitably breaks down or dies, compromising the functional result; therefore, it should be replaced.

In the distal third of the forearm, the ulnar pedicle not only sends branches to the flexor superficialis tendons but also to the skin. These branches are easily identified, being close to the mesotendon branches and of suitable diameter, allowing simultaneously composite transfer of skin and tendon. Generally the skin island lies proximal to the mesotendon position. However, thanks to the pliability and flexibility of these cutaneous branches, the transfer can be rotated and positioned on the digital surface without changing the physiologic direction of tendon fibers. This is of fundamental importance in achieving a good functional result (Figure 4-9).

This new technique, which is now our standard procedure for Boyes class III or IV cases, uses a mesovascular tendon island, and the tendon can be reconstructed in one operation. Compared with all other tendon graft techniques, the advantages of this technique are as follows:

• It makes use of a living tendon island—that of a thin mesotendon with vascular branches, providing a perfect blood supply to all areas, both extrinsic and intrinsic. It thus avoids adhesions and improves the vascularity of the surrounding tissues. Because the transfer is a real flexor tendon and not a simple myotendinous structure, it retains flexibility, pliability, and resistance and allows the correct tension

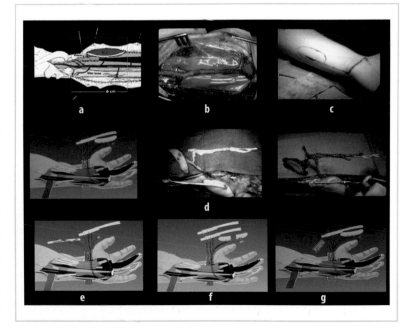

Figure 4-9. a) Diagram of the different vascular branches emerging from the ulnar artery before Guyon's canal entrance. Bone, skin, flexor tendons. **b)** Ulnar artery dissection before Guyon's canal entrance. **c)** A bayonet-shaped incision including an outline of the skin flap is traced on the medial side of the forearm. **d)** Raising of the composite flexor tendon and skin flap island transfer for tendon repair and digital palmar resurfacing. Before and after tourniquet release. **e)** Other multiple combinations: combined island flexor superficialis tendon and palmaris longus transfer for flexor and pulley reconstruction. **f)** The double flexor tendons and double skin flaps transfer. **g)** The composite skin, flexor tendon, and bone transfer. (A.D.F. Video-Productions with special permission)

to be achieved. Because vascularization is preserved, all sheaths are retained. The MVCAS (formerly paratenon) and, in particular, the carpal sheath (which is transposed into "No Man's Land") retain the unrestricted gliding movement of the tendon.

- The tendon transfer is approximately 18 cm to 20 cm long. This length allows easy reconstruction of any type of flexor tendon defect, from the pulp to the carpal area. Thus, the tendon anastomoses are not under tension and lie outside "No Man's Land." Because of the very distal rotation point and the mesotendon plasticity and versatility, placement and anchoring need attention but can be performed without difficulty. The operation is performed in the same way as a classic reversed-flow radial or ulnar forearm flap.

- The mesotendinous vascular branches are anatomically constant, and the dissection will take approximately the same amount of time as a reversed-flow forearm skin flap (approximately 90 minutes).

- This one-stage procedure retains all gliding surfaces, which means that recipient bed preparation by a pseudosynovial sheath using a silicone rod is unnecessary. However, all pulleys have to be repaired carefully: the traction exerted by this type of tendon is greater because the resistance is less. Compared with the other forearm transfers and their potential for composite transfers, the only one that allows simultaneous transposition of skin, bone, and tendon is the radial forearm flap. However, this flap does not allow transfer of the common carpal sheath and the flexor tendon because the radial pedicle supplies them only at the myotendinous level and its rotation point is too proximal. The new technique of composite transfer is specifically confined to the ulnar vascular system and may be conveniently known as the ulnar trail system.

The main disadvantage of our technique is the need to transect the ulnar pedicle. However, in our experience with more than 450 cases of all varieties of ulnar transfers, no undesirable long-term effects, such as paresthesia or functional deficits, have been encountered 1 year after surgery. It is nevertheless preferable to restore arterial continuity with either a venous graft or a vascular prosthesis 2 mm in diameter.

Results of Tendon Reconstruction

Evaluating the results of complex tendon reconstruction is difficult because the variables are too numerous (age of the patient; procedures used; type of injury; accompanying nerve, bone, or vascular injuries; and especially associated skin problems). We prefer the Tubiana classification system[12] because it is based on proximal interphalangeal joint movement, which in our opinion displays the principal effect of the flexor tendon transfer. The arithmetical addition of degrees between extension and flexion compared with the hypothetical maximum amplitude, which does not distinguish between the metacarpophalangeal joint and the proximal interphalangeal or the distal interphalangeal joints, seems inadequate for this sort of salvage situation. Metacarpophalangeal joint movement is rarely altered substantially.

The principal aim in these cases is to restore effective and useful function, including grip, and especially to restore good proximal interphalangeal joint movement. Our results show that 64% percent of these extreme salvage flexor tendon situations achieved an excellent, very good, or good result and were greatly improved in a single operation. These results have to be compared with an average of 55% in results published for similar cases in series using the two-staged procedure with or without a silicone rod. The technique also produces favorable trophic changes. Finger skin becomes more supple and sensitive, joints are less stiff and are mechanically active, and flexion is improved. All this testifies to good biological recovery.

Our results must be improved by a better understanding of flexor tendon biology and the restored gliding mechanism. This new technique seems to give better functional performance and reduces time lost from work.

We present a completely new approach to flexor tendon reconstruction for major salvage surgery. The use of an island flexor tendon, vascularized through the ulnar mesotendon, with all its gliding surfaces intact, seems to be a major advance in dealing with adhesions and has the added merit of being a one-stage procedure. These types of ulnar vascularized tendon or tendon and skin transfers with multiple applications and good functional results could set a trend in tendon reconstructive surgery.

Even if this new procedure restores function, it cannot be used in some circumstances. For example, it cannot be used when all the other fingers have undergone tenolysis. We also know now the complexity of all the sliding tissue around the tendon and how the tendon and sheath have to be considered together as a sliding unit. Using a complete flexion system composed of the flexor tendon, digital sheath, and all the pulleys apparatus seemed to be the perfect reconstruction.

Human Allotransplant of a Digital Flexor System Vascularized on the Ulnar Pedicle

In light of our experience, the idea of a simultaneous tendon and pulley vascularized allotransplant developed gradually. Nonvascularized homografts of an entire flexor tendon complex, originally performed by E. Peacock, had been reported to produce uneven functional results in several cases. These results were doubtless explained by an immunologic response caused by tendon cell components,[7] although there is little or no antigenicity to the collagen tendon structure. These tendon homografts were nonvascularized, taken from cadavers, and either stored by deep-freezing or preserved in Cialit.

The introduction of cyclosporine in 1980 changed the indications and improved success rates in vascularized allotransplantations. Low, nontoxic maintenance doses were prescribed for these relatively weak antigenicity-response organs.

Knowledge of the specific anatomic structure of the ulnar vascular network, experience in homotendon grafts, the use of low-dose cyclosporine, and the necessity to improve functional results have all combined to produce a successful human vascularized allotransplant of a complete digital system by microsurgery.

Transplantation Technique

The original transplantation procedure, based on our knowledge of the ulnar blood supply of the flexor superficialis, especially of the ring finger, has been performed from a living donor. Some refinements and modifications were adopted for the second case from cadaver donor.

The different branches of the ulnar pedicle in the forearm are identified. Those supplying the skin and connected with the forearm anterior venous superficial network and the flexor tendons are selected.

To avoid opening the digital sheath and thus inducing tendon adhesions, we left the two flexor tendons in place in the digital canal. The superficial arcade is clamped and transected between the third and fourth common palmar digital arteries. The functional unit, composed of the flexor tendons and the entire pulley system, is then separated from the digital bone skeleton. This dissection is made in the subperiosteal plane along the skeleton of proximal middle, and distal phalanx. The tendon sheath is not opened. The collateral pedicle is included in the transfer. The ulnar pedicle is ligated above the branch supplying the skin and connected with the venous superficial network (Figure 4-10).

Very good functional results were apparent after 4 months. Wrist swelling disappeared little by little, and because the patient had no active motion preoperatively, the functional result with a range of motion in flexion of 80° in the proximal interphalangeal joint, no extension defect, and 55° of flexion in the distal interphalangeal joint with an extension defect of 35° was considered excellent.

The average total active flexion equalled almost the range of passive motion available. This finger is now very functional and perfectly adapted.

Conclusion

The presented technique is a step toward a new type of reconstruction in hand surgery. It can be used not only for the flexor system, but also for bone and joints. For the moment, medicolegal constraints are severe, and exacting criteria must be met before any transplant can be performed. Such constraints may diminish over time, and techniques of repair and reconstruction, such as those described here, will develop freely for use in selected patients. Despite the success of this technique, it should be reserved for complex cases in which conventional techniques are not possible.

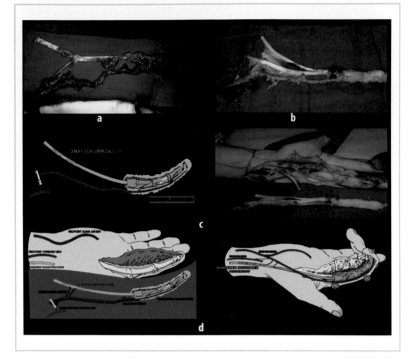

Figure 4-10. Flexor tendon unit allotransplantation program. **a**) A monoflexor superficialis allotransplant after tourniquet release. **b**) A bi flexor superficialis and profundus allotransplant after milking and washing, to be placed in a sterile refrigerated container. **c**) Layout of the allotransplant before inserting. **d**) Insertion and anastomoses. (A.D.F. Video-Productions with special permission)

References

1. Smith JW, Bellinger CG. La vascularisation des tendons. In: Tubiana R, editor. *Traité de la Chirurgie de la Main, Vol. I.* Paris: Masson, 1986.
2. Schatzker J, Branemark PI. Intravital observation on the microvascular anatomy and microcirculation of the tendon. *Acta Orthop Scand.* 1969;126 suppl:1–23.
3. Lundborg G, Myrhage R, Rydevik B. The vascularization of human flexor tendons, the digital synovial sheath region: structural and functional aspects. *J Hand Surg.* 1977;2:417–427.
4. Guimberteau JC. *New Ideas in Hand Flexor Tendon Surgery.* Bordeaux: Ed. Institut Aquitain de la Main, 2001.
5. Guimberteau JC, Sentucq-Rigall J, Panconi B, Boileau R, Mouton P, Bakhach J. Introduction to the knowledge of subcutaneous sliding system in humans. *Ann Chir Plast Esthét.* 2005;50(1):19–34.
6. Guimberteau JC, Delage J, Morlier P. Journey to the tendon and satellite sheath areas; in vivo anatomical observations of flexor tendon vascularization and surrounding sheaths Videofilm, 34 min. Brussels International Symposium: Tendon Lesions, Injuries and Repair. Genval-Brussels, Belgium, 1999. http://www.guimberteau-jc-md.com
7. Guimberteau JC . *Strolling under the skin.* Paris: Elsevier, 2004.
8. Ingber DE. Cellular tensegrity: defining new rules of biological design that govern the cytoskeleton. *J Cell Sci.* 1993;104(3):613–627.
9. D'Arcy Wenworth-Thompson. *On Growth and Form.* (1917). Cambridge: Cambridge University Press, 1961, 1992.
10. Guimberteau JC, Goin JL, Panconi B, Schumacher B. The reverse ulnar artery forearm island flap in hand surgery: about 54 cases. *Plast Reconstr Surg.* 1988;81: 925.
11. Guimberteau JC, Panconi B, Boileau R. Mesovascularized island flexor tendon: new concepts and techniques for flexor tendon salvage surgery. *Plast Reconstr Surg.* 1993;92:888–903.
12. Tubiana R, editor. *Traité de la Chirurgie de la Main, Vol. III.* Paris: Masson,1986.
13. Guimberteau JC, Baudet J, Panconi B, Boileau R, Potaux L. Human allotransplant of a digital flexion system vascularized on the ulnar pedicle: A preliminary report and 1 year follow-up of two cases. *Plast Reconstr J.* 1992;89(6):1135–1147.

5

Innovations in Peripheral Nerve Surgery

Christopher T. Maloney, Jr. and A. Lee Dellon

Introduction

Any talk of innovation in peripheral nerve surgery presupposes the existence of a specialized area of surgery related to the peripheral nerves. With the founding of the American Society for Peripheral Nerve in 1990, and its annual meetings being held in conjunction with the American Association of Hand Surgery and the American Society of Reconstructive Microsurgery, the field of peripheral nerve surgery is clearly now accepted as a specialized field of surgery, with its own body of knowledge.

It has been suggested that James Learmonth, MD, a neurosurgeon from Scotland, should be considered as the pioneer, if not the first, peripheral nerve surgeon.[1] If that suggestion is accepted, then "innovation" in peripheral nerve surgery would be related to the concepts Learmonth introduced. Among these would be the description of surgical techniques, such as decompressing the peripheral nerves, the median nerve compression at the wrist,[2] and the submuscular transposition of the ulnar nerve for compression of the ulnar nerve in the cubital tunnel.[3] Learmonth also described variations in peripheral nerves,[4] the function of peripheral nerves, like the sympathetic nerves,[5] and the idea that a peripheral nerve could be resected to treat pain.[6] In line with these concepts, then, "innovation" will be considered as ideas that lead to new surgical procedures related to the peripheral nerve, whether these new procedures build on earlier descriptions of neuroanatomy or on earlier procedures that have been placed now on a firm evidence base.

"Innovation" also implies "new," and for the purposes of this chapter, the time-line will be within the last 5 years. The concepts that fit into this definition are 1) treating the symptoms of neuropathy by decompressing peripheral nerves, 2) treating long nerve grafts with an allograft, 3) treating short nerve gaps with a conduit, and 4) partial joint denervation for relieving pain, emphasizing the knee, ankle, and shoulder.

Decompressing Nerves to Treat Symptomatic Neuropathy

The hypothesis that the symptoms of neuropathy could be treated by decompressing a peripheral nerve was offered in 1988[7] and supported in a diabetic rat model in 1991[8] and 1994.[9] This hypothesis was confirmed by a separate team in 2003 in the rat model and included the finding that intraneural neurolysis was of added value in improving gait.[10] The hypothesis was confirmed yet again in 2005 in the same model, but this time findings included information specifically on the common peroneal nerve and the gastrocnemius muscle.[11] The first clinical report of the application of these concepts to patients with symptomatic diabetic neuropathy was in 1992,[12] and this application has been confirmed by groups from general surgery in 1995,[13] plastic surgery in 2000[14,15] and 2001,[16] podiatric foot and ankle surgery in 2003,[17] orthopedic foot and ankle surgery in 2004,[18] and neurosurgery in 2004.[19]

At the core of this concept is that the neuropathy itself renders the peripheral nerve susceptible to compression. This fact was documented for diabetes in the streptozotocin rat model in 1988.[20] In the presence of a positive Tinel sign and an appropriate history, carpal tunnel decompression could be done for patients with diabetes and median nerve symptoms. Compression of the median nerve at the wrist, the ulnar nerve at the elbow, and the radial sensory nerve in the forearm conceptually give the physical findings and symptoms of a distal sensory neuropathy—a "glove distribution"—but would be related to three separate nerve compressions. However, in the patient with diabetes, whose nerves are susceptible to compression, these three separate "mononeuropathies" can coexist. Applying this concept to the legs identifies compression of the common peroneal nerve at the knee, the deep peroneal nerve over the dorsum of the foot, and the tibial nerve in the four medial ankle tunnels (not just the tarsal tunnel). A positive Tinel sign over the tibial nerve at the medial ankle has a positive predictive value of 92% in identifying the patient with diabetes who would obtain relief from pain and recovery of sensibility if the four medial ankle tunnels were decompressed (Table 5-1).[21]

In a retrospective series of 50 patients, no ulcerations or amputations occurred during a mean follow-up of 4.5 years after nerve decompression, whereas, ulcerations (n = 12) and amputations (n = 3) did occur in the contralateral leg in which no nerve was decompressed.[22] This difference established that *the natural history of diabetic neuropathy can be changed by decompressing the peripheral nerves in the leg.* Three reviews of this subject appeared early in 2004.[18,23,24] The International Neuropathy Decompression Registry (neuropathyregistry. com), represents a multicenter prospective study with patients being included for decompression if they have 1) neuropathy, 2) a positive Tinel sign over the expected site of nerve entrapment, 3) failed medical management, and 4) surgical

decompression as described by Dellon[25-29] of the common peroneal nerve at the knee, the deep peroneal nerve at the dorsum of the foot, the tarsal tunnel, the medial and lateral plantar tunnels, or the calcaneal tunnel (Figure 5-1).

This concept of decompression was extended to chemotherapy-induced neuropathy based on a rat model of cisplatin neuropathy in 2001.[30] The first patients with chemotherapy-induced neuropathy secondary to cisplatin and Taxol were treated with decompression in 2004.[31] This first report contains just 8 patients. All had relief of pain and recovery of sensation from decompression of upper and lower extremity nerves. Chemotherapy regimens that contain vincristine; platin compounds, such as cisplatin or carboplatin; taxol; or thalidomide can cause a sensory neuropathy that is typically distal and symmetrical, like diabetic neuropathy. This neuropathy is often painful. For cisplatin and Taxol, the peripheral nerve is susceptible to compression by the binding of the chemotherapeutic agent to tubulin in the nerve's axoplasm, which decreases the slow component of anterograde transport. The pain may be severe enough for the patient to stop chemotherapy, at which time nerve decompression would be appropriate. For other patients, neuropathy symptoms, which are dose-related, may improve after cessation of chemotherapy. If the symptoms persist and are disabling, a positive Tinel sign identifies the location of the peripheral nerve compression site. Operative procedures in the leg for chemotherapy-induced neuropathy are the same as those for diabetic neuropathy patients.

The first report of decompression in patients with neuropathy of unknown cause was in 2004.[21] Neuropathy of unknown cause is defined as a distal, diffuse, large-fiber, symmetric neuropathy and it is essentially the same as the type for which pain is relieved and sensibility is restored for patients with diabetic neuropathy, as described above and in Table 5-1. Two more studies were presented at meetings in 2004[19] and in 2005[32] relative to this group of patients with neuropathy of unknown cause (Table 5-2). This subgroup of patients is also reported at the Web site given above.

Outcomes related to decompression of peripheral nerves in patients with symptoms are related in the short term to relief of pain and improvement in sensation (Table 5-1). Secondary outcomes were related to decreased pain and medication and therefore to decreases in the cost of that

Table 5-1. Results of Studies Treating Diabetic Neuropathy with Posterior Tibial Nerve Decompression

Study	Patients (n)	Nerves (n)	Patients Improved (%) Pain	Patients Improved (%) Sensibility
1992, Dellon[12]	31	32	85	72
1995, Wieman[13]	33	26	92	72
2000, Caffee[14]	58	36	86	50
2000, Aszmann[15]	16	12	NA	69
2001, Tambwekr[16]	10	10	80	70
2003, Wood[17]	33	33	90	70
2004, Biddinger[18]	15	22	86	80
2004, Valdivia[19]	60	60	85	85
2004, Lee[29]	46	46	92	92
2005, Steck[32]	25	25	84	72
2005, Rader[89]	49	49	90	72
Total	376	351	88	78

NA = not available

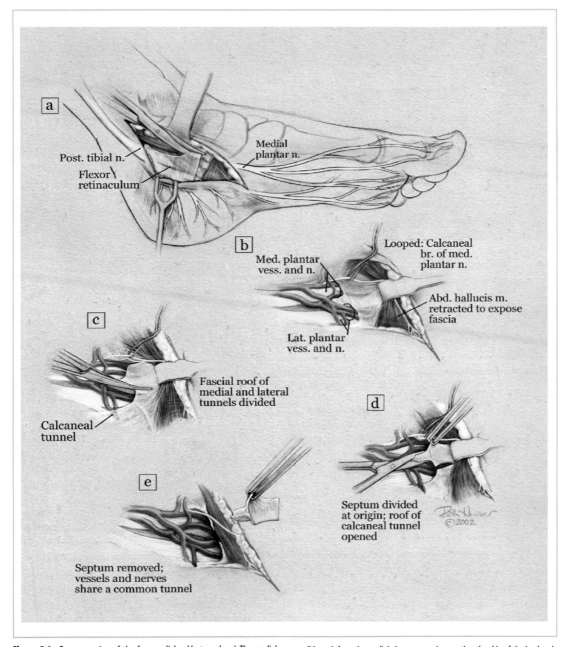

Figure 5-1. Decompression of the four medial ankle tunnels. **a**) The medial ankle region contains the tibial nerve, which passes through four discreet anatomical tunnels, each of which must be decompressed. The tarsal tunnel itself is opened by dividing the flexor retinaculum to expose the tibial vessels and the tibial nerve. In this region, high origins of the calcaneal nerve are identified, and a high division of the tibial nerve is identified, if present. In this region, the tibial nerve is neurolyzed internally, if needed, and sympathetic innervation of the tibial artery can be disrupted. **b**) The abductor hallucis brevis muscle is retracted (not divided) after incising its superficial fascia. In 50% of patients, a small branch from the medial plantar nerve innervating the skin of the heel-arch region is present and is preserved. When the muscle is retracted, the thick fascia providing the roof of the medial and lateral plantar tunnels is identified. **c**) The roof of the medial plantar tunnel has been incised, and the roof of the lateral plantar tunnel is being incised. **d**) The septum between the two tunnels has been cauterized and is being incised to permit the removal of this "T" shaped structure, releasing the medial and lateral plantar nerves into the plantar aspect (porta pedis) of the foot. **e**) The incised calcaneal tunnel is shown, and the "T" structure is being removed.

Table 5-2. Results of Studies Treating Neuropathy of Unknown Cause with Posterior Tibial Nerve Decompression

Study	Patients (n)	Nerves (n)	Patients Improved (%) Pain	Sensibility
2004, Valdivia[19]	40	40	90	80
2004, Lee[21]	40	40	80	80
2005, Steck[32]	26	26	88	68
Total	**106**	**106**	**85**	**72**

medicine. A critical outcome is the change in frequency of ulceration, amputation, or both. This frequency is expected to be 2.3% per year, or a cumulative frequency of 1 of 6 diabetic patients. *None of the studies in Table 5-1 have reported a new ulcer or a new amputation in any of the patients who underwent nerve decompression for symptoms of diabetic neuropathy.* Given that the mean cost of treating a diabetic ulcer was $27,500 in 1998, and that the mean cost for an amputation, including prosthesis, was $40,000, the health care savings of this preventive approach is clear.

Once an ulcer has healed, the recurrence rate in diabetic patients is expected to be between 40% and 60%. From the studies of Wieman and Patel[13] and of Caffee[14] (the only two reports in Table 5-1 in which there were any patients with a history of ulcer or amputation), only 1 of the 29 patients (3%) had a recurrent ulceration. Therefore, even in this advanced population of patients with neuropathy—the subgroup that has a history of ulcer or amputation—restoring sufficient protective sensation to prevent further ulcers saves a substantial amount of money.

This finding supports the results of a recent study in which patients with nerves decompressed in one leg to prevent ulcers experienced ulcers in the other leg, which had the same glycemic control.[22] Therefore, the conclusions from all three experimental studies on diabetic rats[9-11] have been confirmed in clinical studies: in the absence of a site for compression, neuropathy will not occur, and decompression will reverse a neuropathic walking pattern.

A final outcome relates to restoring balance, which prevents falls. Falls in this usually aged population with neuropathy are directly related to loss of balance and commonly result in hip and wrist fractures. There is a direct correlation between loss of sensibility and neuropathy.[33] Restoring sensation to patients with neuropathy by decompressing the peripheral nerves of the leg can improve balance.[34]

Nerve Reconstruction

Two innovations in the treatment of the nerve gap have now been introduced into clinical practice. One is related to treating patients for whom a large nerve graft is needed and for whom this length of graft might not be readily available. This problem has been resolved by nerve allografting. The second innovation is the use of a nerve conduit to connect nerve gaps ranging from those suitable for traditional nerve repair to gaps of up to 3 cm.

Nerve Allografts

Under the leadership of Susan E. Mackinnon, MD, two decades of basic science research have established that 1) the Schwann cells of an allograft are rejected, 2) the host axons regenerate across the basement of the allograft, 3) the host Schwann cells repopulate the reconstructed segment after rejection of the donor Schwann cells, 4) immunosuppression can be discontinued and nerve function preserved after function has been restored, and 5) immunosuppression can be achieved with a regimen less suppressive to the host than that required for kidney or heart-lung or hand transplantation. Current regimens are often based on tacrolimus (FK506) and basiliximab, and a section of nerve is placed subcutaneously to detect rejection.

The first clinical nerve allograft was reported by Mackinnon and Hudson in 1992, for a child with a sciatic nerve injury.[35] That first patient, an 8-year-old boy, was injured in 1988 and required a "10-cable, 23 cm" reconstruction. The first series of nerve allografts, consisting of 7 patients, was reported in 2001.[36] This series included patients with allografts to the arms and legs. In all patients, the nerve gaps and the interposed grafts required constituted a total length of nerve that could not be reconstructed from available host sources. Cadaveric allografts were harvested and preserved for 7 days in University of Wisconsin Cold Storage Solution at 5°C. In the interim, patients were started on an immunosuppressive regimen of either cyclosporin A or FK506, azathioprine, and prednisone. Once sensory or motor function was achieved for 6 months, immunosuppression was stopped. With this approach, 6 of the 7 patients recovered some degree of function, and the one failure was attributed to a "sub-therapeutic" immunosuppressive regimen.

This basic science and clinical research has been done primarily in university hospitals. However, the recent experience of Michael Rose, MD, and Andy Elkwood, MD, plastic surgeons in private practice in southern New Jersey, is relevant. As of January 2005, they had completed five successful nerve allografts (Figure 5-2).[37] Three of their 5 patients received nerve transplants from living-related donors. They received the same regimen as the unrelated donors. Mackinnon's group continues to search for ways to minimize the amount of immunosuppression necessary in nerve allografting. They have described using antibodies to adhesion molecules, modifications of their cold preservation technique, and radiation.[38–40] In time, immunosuppressive regimens that are even less difficult for the patient will be introduced, and patients requiring extensive amounts of peripheral nerve will have their defects reconstructed with nerve allografts. Although perhaps fewer than a dozen clinical nerve allografts have been performed in the past 16 years, this number will increase as other peripheral nerve centers are approved to use this approach to nerve reconstruction.

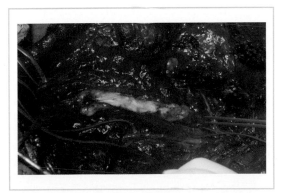

Figure 5-2. Use of nerve allograft to reconstruct a peripheral nerve defect. The pale segment of nerve in the center is the allograft, sutured to the recipient's common peroneal nerve to the right, with connection to the sciatic nerve's common peroneal nerve component to the left. The patient recovered foot dorsiflexion and sensation to the dorsum of the foot. (Courtesy of Michael Rose, MD, and Andrew Elkwood, MD, Short Hills, New Jersey)

Nerve Conduits

More than two decades have passed since experimental models of neural regeneration, using various materials for nerve conduits, were first used to measure neurotrophic substances and to introduce substances related to the nerve regeneration process.[41] Although silicone chambers were among the earliest conduits used experimentally, nerves do not regenerate more than 10 mm in them, primarily because they are nonporous. Furthermore, silicone around a nerve is one model of chronic nerve compression.[42] Nerve regeneration through a region of compression in an animal model does occur, but then the nerve fails, again because of chronic compression.[43]

Silicone has been used for many years to connect nerves that would otherwise have undergone primary repair, but even the most recent report of this approach, in 2004, describes the necessity of removing the silicone from patients as a result of long-term problems with symptoms of compression or pain.[44] The first ever randomized multicenter, blinded study of a nerve conduit for reconstructing a sensory nerve defect in the hand was reported in 2000 by Weber et al.[45] The conduit was a porous, polyglycolic acid (PGA) bioabsorbable conduit that is removed by hydrolysis, called the Neurotube (formerly distributed by Neuroegen, and, as of December of 2004, by Synovis Microsystems). Dellon and Mackinnon first reported the results of neural regeneration through this tube. The results were equivalent to those obtained with standard interposition interfascicular sural nerve grafts in a nonhuman primate to repair a 3-cm ulnar nerve defect at the elbow (with recovery of intrinsic motor function at one year).[46] This 1988 report was followed by the first clinical report of conduit in the sensory nerves in the human hand.[47] The maximum gap for clinical use was established at 3 cm by demonstrating in nonhuman primates that neural regeneration at a greater distance was not successful.[48]

The Neurotube has been successful in treating sensory or mixed nerves in the arms and legs, as well as in cranial nerves V, VII, and XI in humans (Table 5-3). The results of a randomized study, by Weber et al, were that *the Neurotube resulted in statistically significant better recovery of sensation for nerve gaps less than 4 mm and greater*

Table 5-3. Reports of Clinical Applications of the Neurotube

Peripheral Nerve Reconstructed Report	Date of
Sensory Nerve: Arm	
Digital and Median at the Wrist[47]	1990
Digital[45]	2000
Digital[49]	2003
Sensory Nerve: Foot[50]	2001
Cranial Nerves: Sensory	
V (inferior alveoloar)[51]	1992
Cranail Nerve: Motor	
VII (facial)[52]	2005
XI (spinal accessory)[53]	2005

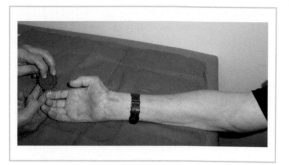

Figure 5-4. Reconstruction of the median and ulnar nerve at the level of the brachium 18 months ago in a 51-year-old man. Note the recovered bulk of the forearm muscles. Electromyographic evidence of reinnervation of the flexor carpi radialis, flexor profundus, flexor superficialis, pronator, and flexor carpi ulnaris was obtained. Sensation was recovered in the fingertips with two-point discrimination and good localization 24 months after the Neurotube reconstruction. Two tubes were placed for the ulnar nerve and three for the median nerve. (Courtesy of A. L. Dellon, MD.)

than 8 mm, indicating that the Neurotube should be the conduit of choice for either a primary repair or a nerve gap reconstruction of less than 30 mm.[45] The Neurotube has been used with

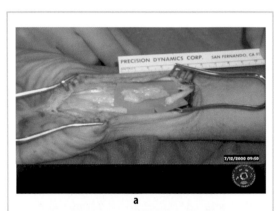

a

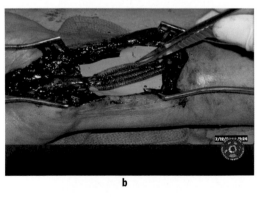

b

Figure 5-3. Reconstruction of the neuroma-in-continuity of the median nerve in the forearm of a 37-year-old man. Previous primary repair was unsuccessful. **a**) Resection of the neuroma showing the 3-cm gap in the median nerve. The tourniquet is inflated. **b**) Interfascicular reconstruction of the defect with four, 2.3-mm-diameter Neurotubes, each 4 cm long.

multiple conduits, instead of multiple sural nerve grafts, to reconstruct the median nerve at the wrist (Figure 5-3), and to reconstruct the median and ulnar nerve in the brachium of the forearm in a 51-year-old man (Figure 5-4).

The Food and Drug Administration approved the Neurotube for clinical use in 1997. After that approval, other conduits could be used without the need for randomized controlled studies in humans. An example of one such tube is the NeuraGen collagen tube by Integra LifeSciences (and not to be confused with the Neurotube, which is made of PGA, amino acid, and sugar molecules, and not a foreign protein). No clinical trials of this collagen tube have yet been published. A series of 9 patients was described at the 2005 meeting of the American Society for Peripheral Nerve Surgery.[54] The collagen is bovine, and as such carries the risk of an inflammatory or immunological reaction, in contrast to the PGA tube, which is hydrolyzed. In this series of patients who received the collagen tube (the size of the nerve gap is not given), the recovery of sensation was described as "at least protective, with the mean static 2-point discrimination being 9 mm." This average result is much inferior to that obtained with the Neurotube, where the mean static 2-point discrimination was 3.7 mm for defects less than 4 mm and 6.8 mm for defects greater than 8 mm.[45]

Another tube available now in the US is made of poly DL-lactide-e-caprolactone (Durolac;

Polyganics BV, Groningen, Netherlands). A series of patients receiving this conduit also was presented at the American Society for Peripheral Nerve meeting in 2005.[54,55] The results with this conduit were *not* better than those with the control repair or graft. There is evidence that portions of this tube remain present for more than 18 months, which is similar to the collagen tube. This presence suggests that the term "bioabsorbable" may not be the best description for these tubes; the PGA tube looses tensile strength by 3 months and then is hydrolyzed relatively quickly. *Another important difference is that the collagen and the Durolac tubes are available in a length of only 2 cm. Because the nerve must occupy the first 5 mm at each end of the tube, only defects less than 1.0 cm can be reconstructed. In contrast, the Neurotube is available in a 4-cm length, which means that a 3-cm defect can be reconstructed.* Given the ability of nerves to regenerate through almost any conduit, more competitive tubes will likely become commercially available for clinical use. At present, only the Neurotube, as established in Table 5-3, offers proven capability for both sensory and motor, extremity and cranial nerve defects for clinical nerve reconstruction.

Partial Joint Denervation

Partial joint denervation is the concept of preserving joint function and relieving joint pain by interrupting the neural pathway that transmits the pain message from the joint to the brain. *Traditional approaches to treating joint pain rely on musculoskeletal approaches to the joint itself and often require joint fusion or total replacement arthroplasty. The concept of partial joint denervation offers the patient an outpatient, ambulatory operative approach that is join — sparing and rehabilitation-free.* Establishing the validity of partial joint denervation requires 1) identifying the innervation of the specific joint through dissection because this information is not contained in anatomy texts, 2) defining a route to administer local anesthetic based on this new anatomic knowledge, 3) demonstrating that local anesthetics will relieve pain in patients in whom the musculoskeletal approach has failed, 4) planning a surgical approach to resect the nerve and interrupting the pain pathway, and 5) documenting the success of this approach with an appropriate patient population. This process must be repeated for each different joint.

Partial joint denervation was introduced by Dellon in a 1978 description of the innervation of the dorsal wrist capsule by the posterior interosseous nerve[56] and in his description of the treatment of pain related to injury to that nerve in 1985.[57] The innervation of the anterior wrist joint was described in 1984, and partial volar wrist denervation was then possible.[58] Before this approach, total wrist denervation had been described and practiced in Europe but required 4 incisions and removal of 10 different nerve branches.[59,60] The extension of the concept of partial joint denervation was then extended by Dellon to the knee joint.[61-63] Through 2000, the reported results for 344 patients treated with partial knee denervation (Table 5-4) are that 90% responded to a local anesthetic block with increased ambulation, stair climbing, kneeling, and reduced pain (improvement of at least 5 mm on a visual analog scale for pain).[69] Causes for less-than-good results were related to

Table 5-4. Partial Joint Denervation: Relationship of Joint to its Innervation

Painful Anatomic Site	Nerve Innervating Site	Denervation Described
Wrist, Dorsal	Posterior interosseous, 1978[56]	Dellon, 1985[57]
Wrist, Volar	anterior interosseous, 1984[58]	Dellon, 1984[58]
Knee	medial & lateral retinacular, 1994[61]	Dellon, 1995[62]
Sinus Tarsi	deep peroneal nerve, 2001[64]	Dellon, 2002[65]
Shoulder, Anterior	lateral thoracic, 1995[66]	Dellon, 2003[67]
Elbow, Lateral Epicondyle	Posterior brachial cutaneous nerve, 1962[83]	DeJesus, 2004[84]
Elbow, Medial Epicondyle	br. to medial epicondyle, 2004[85]	Dellon, 2004[86]
Temporomandibular Joint	auriculotemporal & br. of masseteric, 2003[68]	Dellon, 2005[80]

worker's compensation disability issues and drug addiction. Because of variability in the cutaneous nerves to the knee, about 10% of patients require a second operation to resect another cutaneous nerve, usually from the infrapatellar branch of the saphenous nerve. The experience with this procedure now exceeds 600 patients, and the results are similar (ALD, personal experience). This approach has been extended to other joints (Table 5-4), and its extension to the lateral ankle and shoulder are described below.

O'Conner first described sinus tarsi syndrome in 1958.[70] Lateral ankle (the sinus tarsi) pain is most commonly cause by an inversion sprain. The sinus tarsi are a space related to the bones of the anterolateral ankle (Figures 5-5a and 5-5b). The pain may be associated with a fracture

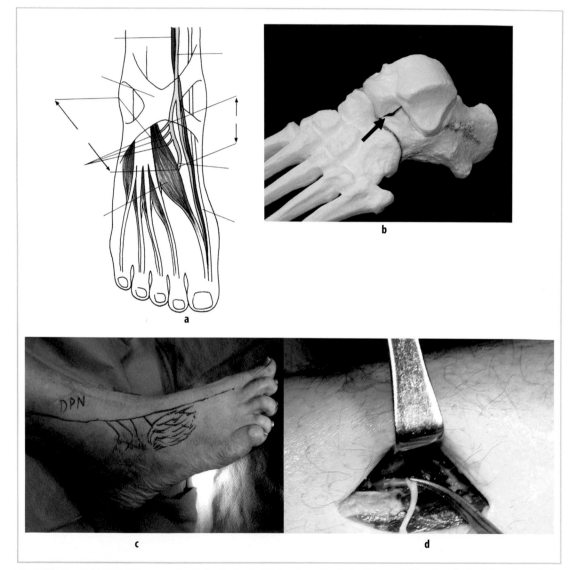

Figure 5-5. The anterolateral ankle has a space described as the sinus tarsi that is illustrated in **a**) and **b**). In **a**), the deep peroneal nerve is shown innervating the extensor brevis muscle, and in **b**), the sinus tarsi is identified by the black arrow. In **c**), the deep peroneal nerve is shown innervating the sinus tarsi proximal to its innervating the brevis. Its terminal branch to the dorsal first webspace is also shown. In **d**), the deep peroneal nerve is resected through an approach in the lateral leg, to denervate the sinus tarsi.

or dislocation, but it is always associated with a tear of the ligaments to the joints in this space. When traditional non-operative treatment for sinus tarsi syndrome fails, and pain becomes recalcitrant, surgical options usually involved evacuating the contents of the sinus tarsi (sometimes referred to as a "clean out"), a subtalar joint arthrodesis, or a subtalar joint arthroscopy.[71–73]

The innervation of the sinus tarsi was described in 2001 as being from the deep peroneal nerve, with the branch(es) arising just proximal to the ankle in 100% of people (Figure 5-5c), and with additional innervation coming from the sural nerve in about 20% of people.[64] The evaluation of these patients requires previous foot and ankle consultation to be sure that all musculoskeletal sources of pain have been treated and that the ankle is strong. This evaluation includes being sure that there are no bone fragments in the subtalar joint. First, nerve blocks with local anesthetic must be done for the deep peroneal nerve proximal to the ankle, and then, if there is still pain with ambulation, the sural nerve should be blocked. Although the first patient reported excellent pain relief after partial resection of the deep peroneal nerve just above the ankle, which preserved function in the extensor brevis muscle and the distal dorsal foot skin,[65] in a larger series, some patients did not experience relief. The current recommendation is to resect the entire deep peroneal nerve through the anterolateral lower leg (Figure

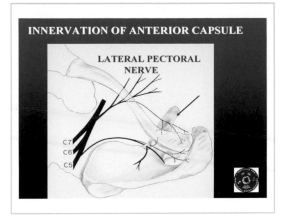

Figure 5-7. Innervation of the anterior shoulder capsule from a branch of the lateral pectoral nerve (arrow). Because this nerve crosses the coracoid, it is the site for a nerve block.

5-5d),[74] as described for the treatment of dorsal foot neuromas.[75] Results obtained with partial resection of the deep peroneal nerve were excellent in 4 patients, good in 2, and poor in 1, in contrast to the results of traditional therapy, which were excellent in 6 and poor in 1 (Figure 5-6).[74] The one failure in this last group of patients involved a complex regional pain syndrome.

Anterior shoulder pain is the most common symptom of failed orthopedic approaches to treating impingement syndrome and rotator cuff tears. Shoulder pain limits movement of the shoulder, the ability to perform activities of daily living, and many work activities, in particular work requiring the overhead use of the hand.

Over the past 25 years, open or arthroscopic approaches to correct shoulder pain has left about 20% of patients with anterior shoulder pain.[76–79] In 1967, a description of the innervation of the anterior shoulder capsule from a branch of the lateral thoracic nerve (Figure 5-7)[67] suggested that this nerve could be blocked by local anesthetic injection on the surface of the coracoid (Figures 5-8a and 5-8b). Before the block, the patient's pain is measured with a visual analog scale, and the range of painless shoulder motion is identified. The nerve is then blocked, taking care not to inject too deeply to the coracoid, to prevent blocking the brachial plexus and injuring the lung. If the block is successful, within 10 minutes the patient's pain will diminish and range of motion of the shoulder will improve (Figures 5-8c and 5-8d).

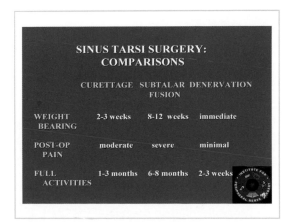

Figure 5-6. Characteristics of recovery from different surgeries for sinus tarsi syndrome.

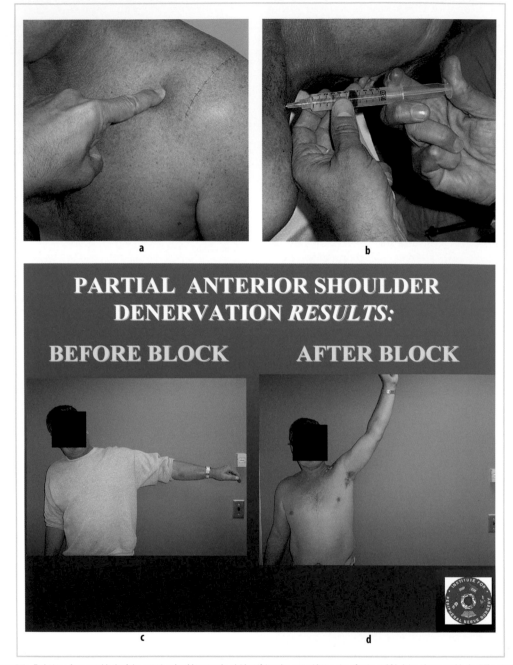

Figure 5-8. Technique for nerve block of the anterior shoulder capsule. **a**) Identifying the coracoid as a site of pain and **b**) doing the nerve block. **c**) The site before surgery and **d**) after a successful block, establishing that this nerve was the source of shoulder pain.

Residual impairment in the range of motion may remain as a result of adhesive capsulitis. If the denervation procedure is successful, subsequent surgery can improve the range of motion of the "frozen shoulder." The incision is made over the coracoid, and the pectoralis muscle is split longitudinally (Figure 5-9a). Loup magnification and bipolar coagulation is used. The vessels in the loose areolar tissue just deep to the pectoralis and immediately over the coracoid

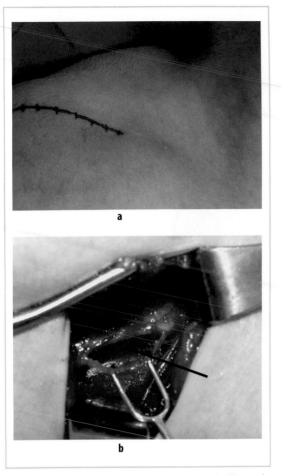

a

b

Figure 5-9. Intra-operative view of a nerve to the anterior shoulder capsule. **a)** The incision on the right shoulder of a patient who had a previous open-shoulder surgery. **b)** A nerve to the anterior shoulder capsule adjacent to vessels.

are inspected, and any nerve within this tissue is excised, often requiring excision of one of the veins as well (Figure 5-9b). Then, the coracoid is approached, and the origin of the biceps and coracobrachialis inspected. A second branch of the nerve may be present at this level, measuring less than 1.0 mm. A 2-cm segment is resected. Marcaine is placed into this area. If there is any question about the nerve being a motor branch to the pectoralis, intra-operative stimulation is used. The nerve typically can be traced directly to the shoulder capsule, but it is resected over the coracoid.

The results in the first group of 12 patients treated with this technique were reported in 2003, to the Argentinian Hand Surgery Society meeting (Figure 5-10).[67] The mean age of the 8 men and 4 women was 37.5 years (range 29 to 54 years). The mechanism of injury was work-related in 7. The mean time from injury to shoulder denervation was 2.5 years (range: 0.5 to 7.0 years). To be eligible for the procedure, each patient had to have at least 5 points on the pain scale and required an increase in range of motion. At a mean of 1.2 years after anterior shoulder denervation, 8 patients had excellent results and 4 had good results. Mean VAS pain scores dropped from 8.5 to 1.8, and mean range of motion, pain-free, increased from 0° to 60° to 1° to 100°.

Elbow joint pain must be distinguished from medial and lateral humeral epicondylar pain. Although the innervation of the elbow joint was described more than half a century ago,[80] and total elbow denervation was described more than 40 years ago,[81,82] partial elbow joint denervation has not been described, nor has isolated denervation of either the medial or lateral humeral epicondyle. Kaplan and Wilhelm did describe denervation of the lateral humeral epicondylitis, but Kaplan[81] clearly denervated only branches of the radial nerve at the radial-humeral joint, whereas Wilhelm[82] did this as well, plus denervating muscles innervated at the epicondyle. He also included the posterior brachial cutaneous nerve (nervus cutaneous antebrachii dorsalis) in perhaps his first description of this procedure in German, in 1962.[83]

In 2004, isolated denervation of the lateral humeral epicondyle by resecting the branches of the posterior cutaneous nerve of the arm and forearm was described at the American Association of Hand Surgery meeting.[84] The innervation of the medial humeral epicondyle was described in 2005 at the American Society for Peripheral Nerve. This nerve was noted during resection of the medial intermuscular septum during submuscular transposition of the ulnar nerve. Cadaver dissections revealed that it originates from the radial nerve in the axilla in all cases, with one case having a contribution from the ulnar nerve in the axilla as well. This nerve can be resected at the insertion of the medial intermuscular septum into the medial epicondyle for the treatment of medial epicondylitis ("golfer's elbow").[85,86]

Temporomandibular joint (TMJ) pain is another example of debilitating joint pain.

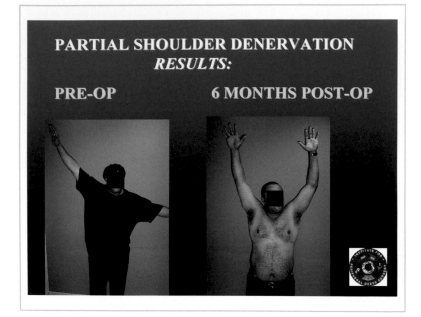

Figure 5-10. Results of anterior shoulder denervation. A typical patient preoperatively and 6 months after surgery, showing increased range of motion.

Although TMJ pain is taught traditionally to be related to dental malocclusion, it if often considered to be part of the symptom complex in brachial plexus compression, in the thoracic inlet (thoracic outlet syndrome) and cervical sprain. The TMJ can be the center of referred pain from the cervical plexus, as in the two clinical examples given above, from the maxillary sinusitis (infraorbital nerve), or from third molar problems (superior and inferior alveolar nerves). This referral pattern is best understood by relating it to the recent iteration of the many earlier papers that describe the innervation of the TMJ, from branches of the trigeminal nerve division V2, the mandibular nerve. The lateral aspect of the TMJ is innervated by the auriculotemporal nerve before it pierces the temporal fascia to innervate the preauricular and temporal region. The medial aspect of the TMJ is innervated by a branch from the nerve that innervates the masseter muscle just before that nerves crosses between the coronoid and condylar processes, at the mandibular notch.[68] Additional medial innervation may come from the nerve to the lateral pterygoid muscle.[68]

Despite extensive protocols for managing TMJ pain, if they fail, endoscopic or open procedures attempt to tighten the ligaments of the TMJ or to reshape or reconstruct the joint itself. These procedures classically give immediate relief, but pain recurs in 3 to 6 months. Much of this success is likely related to completely denervating the TMJ, and the recurring pain is caused by reinnervation of the joint or true neuroma formation.

On January 28, 2005, the first attempt to denervate the TMJ was performed (Figure 5-11a) in a patient who had three previous procedures, two endoscopic and one open.[87] A preauricular incision was made, and the upper portion of the mandibular ramus was approached, using a dilute epinephrine solution to control bleeding and intraoperative electrical stimulation to identify the facial nerve branches (Figure 5-11b). The auriculotemporal nerve moves from posterior to anterior across this portion of the mandible and may be identified at this point (Figure 5-11b) and followed to the lateral TMJ capsule, and resected (Figure 5-11c). A branch to the eustachian tube can be identified and should also be resected because this branch may create referred or neuromatous pain in the external auditory meatus (which it did in this patient, preventing her from wearing her hearing aid). The branch from the nerve to the masseter is difficult to identify, but it was approached in this patient by extending the incision toward the mandibular

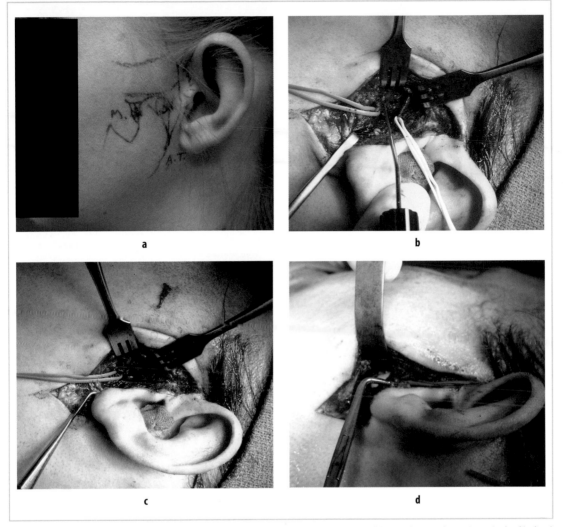

a

b

c

d

Figure 5-11. Denervation of the temporomandibular joint (TMJ). **a**) Preoperative view of the TMJ outlined with innervation, from the auriculotemporal nerve to the lateral and the masseteric nerve to the medial side of the joint capsule. **b**) Intra-operative view, with the blue vessel loop on a facial nerve branch (note nerve stimulator in use) and white vessel loop on branch of auriculotemporal nerve. **c**) After resection of the auriculotemporal nerve, its proximal end is placed deep to the mandibular ramus (dark hole and arrow). The specimen is lying on the cheek skin. **d**) The branch of the masseteric nerve to the joint capsule is approached by elevating the masseter from the mandibular ramus (white area) and then grasping the nerve with a right-angle clamp, reaching behind the condyle.

angle, elevating the masseter from the mandible, and dissecting superiorly towards the notch. In this location, a right angle clamp can be placed posteriorly, and the innervation of the medial TMJ can be disrupted (Figure 5-11c). It may be that only a partial, lateral TMJ denervation is needed for most patients with intractable TMJ pain.

For plastic surgery, the concept of partial joint denervation opens a new area for patient care, permitting relief of pain and restoration of

function throughout the body for those with joint pain.

References

1. Dellon AL, Amadio PC, James R. Learmonth: the first peripheral nerve surgeon. *J Reconstr Microsurg*. 2000; 16:213–216.
2. Learmonth JR. The principle of decompression in the treatment of certain disease of peripheral nerves. *Surg Clin North Am*. 1933;13:905–913.

3. Learmonth JR. Technique for transplanting the ulnar nerve. *Surg Gyn Obst.* 1942;75:792–793.

4. Learmonth JR. A variation in the distribution of the radial branch of the musculo spiral nerve. *J Anat.* 1918; 53:371–374.

5. Learmonth JR, Markowitz J. Studies on the function of the lumbar sympathetic outflow. I. The relation of the lumbar sympathetic outflow to the sphincter ani internus. *Am J Physiol.* 1929;89:686–691.

6. Learmonth JR, Montgomery H, Counseller VS. Resection of sensory nerves of perineum in certain irritative conditions of the external genitalia. *Arch Surg.* 1933; 26:50–63.

7. Dellon AL. Optimism in diabetic neuropathy. *Ann Plast Surg.* 1988;20:103–105.

8. Dellon ES, Dellon AL. Functional assessment of neurologic impairment: track analysis in diabetic and compression neuropathies. *Plast Reconstr Surg.* 1991; 88:686–694.

9. Dellon ES, Dellon AL, Seiler WA IV. The effect of tarsal tunnel decompression in the streptozotocin-induced diabetic rat. *Microsurg.* 1994;15:265–268.

10. Kale B, Yuksel F, Celikoz B, Sirvanci S, Ergun O, Arbak S. Effect of various nerve decompression procedures on the functions of distal limbs in streptozotocin induced diabetic rats: further optimism in diabetic neuropathy. *Plast Reconstr Surg.* 2003;111:2265–2272.

11. Demir Y, Sari A, Siemionow M. Impact of early decompression on development of superimposed neuropathy in diabetic rats. Paper presented at the American Association for Surgery of the Hand annual meeting, Puerto Rico, January 15, 2005.

12. Dellon AL. Treatment of symptoms of diabetic neuropathy by peripheral nerve decompression. *Plast Reconstr Surg.* 1992;89:689–697.

13. Wieman TJ, Patel VG. Treatment of hyperesthetic neuropathic pain in diabetics; decompression of the tarsal tunnel. *Ann Surg.* 1995;221:660–665.

14. Chafee H. Decompression of peripheral nerves for diabetic neuropathy. *Plast Reconstr Surg.* 2000;106: 813–815.

15. Aszmann OA, Kress KM, Dellon AL. Results of decompression of peripheral nerves in diabetics: a prospective, blinded study *Plast Reconstr Surg.* 2000: 106:816–821.

16. Tambwekar SR. Extended neurolysis of the posterior tibial nerve to improve sensation in diabetic neuropathic feet. *Plast Reconstr Surg.* 2001;108:1452–1453.

17. Wood WA, Wood MA. Decompression of peripheral nerve for diabetic neuropathy in the lower extremity. *J Foot Ankle Surg.* 2003;42:268–275.

18. Biddinger K, Amend KA. The role of surgical decompression for diabetic neuropathy. *Foot Ankle Clin N Am.* 2004;9:239–254.

19. Valdivia JMV, Weinand M, Maloney CT Jr. Surgical treatment of peripheral neuropathy: outcomes from 100 consecutive surgical cases. Paper presented at the Neurosurgical Society of the Southwest annual meeting, Phoenix, AZ, 2004.

20. Dellon AL, Mackinnon SE, Seiler WA IV. Susceptibility of the diabetic nerve to chronic compression. *Ann Plast Surg.* 1988;20:117–119.

21. Lee C, Dellon AL. Prognostic ability of Tinel sign in determining outcome for decompression surgery in diabetic and non-diabetic neuropathy. *Ann Plast Surg.* 2004;53:523–527.

22. Aszmann OC, Tassler PL, Dellon AL. Changing the natural history of diabetic neuropathy: incidence of ulcer/amputation in the contralateral limb of patients with a unilateral nerve decompression procedure. *Ann Plast Surg.* 2004;53:517–522.

23. Siemionow M, Demir Y. Diabetic neuropathy: pathogenesis and treatment. A Review. *J Reconstr Micros.* 2004; 20:241–252.

24. Dellon AL. Review of surgical approach to restore sensation, relieve pain, prevent ulcer and prevent amputation. *Foot Ankle Int.* 2004;25:749–755.

25. Mackinnon SE, Dellon AL. Homologies between the tarsal and carpal tunnels: implications for treatment of the tarsal tunnel syndrome. *Contemp Orthop.* 1987;14: 75–79.

26. Mackinnon SE, Dellon AL. *Surgery of the Peripheral Nerve.* New York: Thieme, 1988.

27. Dellon AL. Entrapment of the deep peroneal nerve on the dorsum of the foot. *Foot Ankle.* 1990;11:73–80.

28. Dellon AL. Computer-assisted sensibility evaluation and surgical treatment of tarsal tunnel syndrome. *Adv Pod.* 1996;2:17–40.

29. Dellon AL, Ebmer J, Swier P. Anatomic variations related to decompression of the common peroneal nerve at the fibular head. *Ann Plast Surg.* 2002;48:30–33.

30. Tassler PL, Dellon AL, Lesser G, Grossman S. Utility of decompressive surgery in the prophylaxis and treatment of cisplatin neuropathy in adult rats. *J Reconstr Surg.* 2000;16:457–463.

31. Dellon AL, Swier P, Levingood M, Maloney CT. Cisplatin/Taxol neuropathy: treatment by decompression of peripheral nerve. *Plast Reconstr Surg.* 2004;114: 478–483.

32. Steck JK. Results of decompression of lower extremity nerves in patients with symptomatic neuropathy of unknown etiology. Paper presented at the American Society for Peripheral Nerve annual meeting, Puerto Rico, January 16, 2005.

33. Ducic I, Dellon AL, Short KW. Relationship between loss of pedal sensibility, balance, and falls in patients with peripheral neuropathy. *Annals Plast Surg.* 2004;52: 535–540.

34. Ducic I, Taylor N, Dellon AL. Relationship between peripheral nerve decompression and gain of pedal sensibility and balance in patients with peripheral neuropathy. Paper presented at the American Society for Peripheral Nerve annual meeting, Puerto Rico, January 16, 2005.

35. Mackinnon SE, Hudson AR. Clinical application of peripheral nerve transplantation. *Plast Reconstr Surg.* 1992;90:695–699.

36. Mackinnon SE, Doolabh VG, Novak CB, Trulock EP. Clinical outcome following nerve allograft transplantation. *Plast Reconstr Surg.* 2001;107:1419–1429.

37. Rose M. Our experience with nerve allografting in private practice. Paper presented at the Institute for Peripheral Nerve Surgery Fellowship Group meeting, Lake Las Vegas, NV, September 2004.

38. Tung TH, Doolabh VB, Mackinnon SE, Hunter DA, Flye MW. Immune unresponsiveness by intraportal UV-B irradiated donor antigen administration requires persistence of donor antigen in a nerve allograft model. *J Reconstr Microsurg.* 2004;20:43–51.

39. Brenner MJ, Jensen JN, Lowe JB III, Myckatyn TM, Fok IK, Hunder DA, et al. Anti-CD40 ligand antibody permits regeneration through peripheral nerve allografts in a

nonhuman primate model. *Plast Reconstruc Surg.* 2004; 114:1802–1814.

40. Fox IK, Jaramillo A, Hunter DA, Rickman SR, Mohanakumar T, Mackinnon SE. Prolonged cold-preservation of nerve allografts. *Muscle Nerve.* 2005;31:59–69.

41. Longo FM, Manthorpe M, Skaper SD, Lundborg G, Varon S. Neuronotropic activities accumulate in vivo within silicone nerve regeneration chambers. *Brain Res.* 1983;261:109–117.

42. Mackinnon SE, Dellon AL, Hudson AR, Hunter DA. A primate model for chronic nerve compression. *J Reconstr Microsurg.* 1985;1:185–194.

43. Johnston B, Zachary LS, Dellon AL, Mackinnon SE. Neural regeneration through a distal site of nerve compression. *J Reconstr Microsurg.* 1993;9:271–274.

44. Lundborg G, Rosen B, Dahlin L, Holmberg J, Rosen I. Tubular repair of the median or ulnar nerve in the human forearm: a 5-year follow-up. *J Hand Surg.* 2004; 29B:100–107.

45. Weber RA, Breidenbach WC, Brown RE, Jabaley ME, et al. A randomized prospective study of polyglycolic acid conduits for digital nerve reconstruction in humans. *Plast Reconstr Surg.* 2000;106:1036–1045.

46. Dellon AL, Mackinnon SE. An alternative to the classical nerve graft for the management of the short nerve gap. *Plast Reconstr Surg.* 1988;82:849–856.

47. Mackinnon SE, Dellon AL. Clinical nerve reconstruction with a bioabsorbable polyglycolic acid tube. *Plast Reconstr Surg.* 1990;85:419–424.

48. Mackinnon SE, Dellon AL. A study of nerve regeneration across synthetic (Maxon) and biological (collagen) nerve conduits for nerve gaps up to 5 cm in the primate. *J Reconstr Microsurg.* 1990;6:117–121.

49. Laroas G, Battiston G, Sard A, Ferrero M, Dellon AL. Digital nerve reconstruction with the bioabsorbable Neurotube. *Clinical Exper Plastic Surg.* 2003;35: 125–128.

50. Kim J, Dellon AL. Reconstruction of a painful post-traumatic medial plantar neuroma with a bioabsorbable nerve conduit: a case report. *J Foot Ankle Surg.* 2001; 40:318–323.

51. Crawley WA, Dellon AL. Inferior alveolar nerve reconstruction with a polyglycolic acid, bioabsorbable nerve conduit: a case report. *Plast Reconstr Surg.* 1992;90:300–302.

52. Navaro M, Battiston B. Facial nerve function restored with the Neurotube for acute facial nerve injuries. *Brit J Plast Surg.* In press.

53. Ducic I, Maloney CT, Dellon AL. Reconstruction of the spinal accessory nerve with autograft or Neurotube? two case reports. *J Reconstr Microsurg.* 2005;21:29–33.

54. Bindra R, Sager BJ, Betts K. Use of a collagen conduit for primary repair of complex digital nerve injuries. Paper presented at the American Society for Peripheral Nerve annual meeting, Puerto Rico, 2005.

55. Meek MF, Bertleff MJOE, Ritt MJPF, Van der Lei B, De Boer A, Houpt P, et al. A randomized prospective multicenter study of a biodegradable Neurolac® nerve guide for sensory nerve repair in the hand. Paper presented at the American Society for Peripheral Nerve annual meeting, Puerto Rico, 2005.

56. Dellon AL, Seif SS. Neuroma of the posterior interosseous nerve simulating a recurrent ganglion: case report and anatomical dissection relating the posterior interosseous nerve to the carpus and etiology of dorsal ganglion pain. *J Hand Surg.* 1978;3:326–332.

57. Dellon AL. Partial dorsal wrist denervation: resection of distal posterior interosseous nerve. *J Hand Surg.* 1985; 10A:527–533.

58. Dellon AL, Mackinnon SE, Daneshvar A. Terminal branch of anterior interosseous nerve as source of wrist pain. *J Hand Surg.* 1984;19B:316–322.

59. Wilhelm A. Zur Entwicklungsgeschichte der Gelenke der oberen Extremität [German]. *Z Anat und Entwicklungsgesch.* 1958;120:331–371.

60. Buck-Gramcko D. Denervation of the wrist joint. *J Hand Surg.* 1977;2A:54–61.

61. Horner G, Dellon AL. Innervation of the human knee joint and implications for surgery. *Clin Orthop Rel Res.* 1994;301:221–226.

62. Dellon AL, Mont MA, Hungerford DS. Partial denervation for treatment of persistent neuroma pain after total knee arthroplasty. *Clin Orthop Rel Res.* 1995;316:145–150.

63. Dellon AL, Mont M, Mullik T, Hungerford D. Partial denervation for persistent neuroma pain around the knee. *Clin Orthop Rel Res.* 1996;329:216–222.

64. Rab M, Ebmer J, Dellon AL. Innervation of the sinus tarsi: implications for treating anterolateral ankle pain. *Ann Plastic Surg.* 2001;47:500–504.

65. Dellon AL. Denervation of the sinus tarsi for chronic post-traumatic lateral ankle pain. *Orthopedics.* 2002;25: 849–851.

66. Aszmann OC, Dellon AL, Birely B, McFarland E. Innervation of the human shoulder joint and its implications for surgery. *Clin Orthop Rel Res.* 1996;330: 202–207.

67. Dellon AL. Denervation of the anterior shoulder joint. Paper presented at the Argentinian Hand Surgery Society meeting, Buenos Aires, Argentina, 2003.

68. Davidson JA, Metzinger SE, Tufaro AP, Dellon AL. Innervation of the temporomandibular joint. *J Craniofacial Surg.* 2003;14:235–239.

69. Dellon AL, Mont MA, Hungerford DS. Partial denervation for the treatment of painful neuromas complicating total knee arthroplasty. In: Insall JN, Scott WN, editors. *Surgery of the Knee.* Philadelphia: W.B. Saunders Co., 2000:1772–1786.

70. O'Conner D. Sinus Tarsi Syndrome. A Clinical Entity. *J Bone Joint Surg.* 1958;40A:720.

71. Canale ST. Ankle injuries. In: *Campbell's Operative Orthopedics,* Vol. 2, 9th ed., 1998:1096–1097.

72. Boberg J, Kalish SR, Banks AS. Ankle conditions. In: *McGlamery's Comprehensive Textbook of Foot Surgery,* Vol. 1. Philadelphia: Lippincott Williams & Wilkins, 1987.

73. Olaff LM, Schulhofer SD, Bocko AP. Subtalar joint arthroscopy for sinus tarsi syndrome: a review of 29 cases. *J Foot Ankle Surg.* 2001;40:152–157.

74. Barrett S, Dellon AL. Denervation of the sinus tarsi. *J Amer Pod Med Assoc.* In press.

75. Dellon AL, Aszmann OC. Treatment of dorsal foot neuromas by translocation of nerves into anterolateral compartment. *Foot Ankle.* 1998;19:300–303.

76. Rowe CR, Patel D, Southmayd WW. The Bankart procedure. *J Bone Joint Surg.* 1978;60A:1–16.

77. Ellman H, Hanker G, Bayer M. Repair of the rotator cuff: end-result study of factors influencing reconstruction. *J Bone Joint Surg.* 1986;68A:1136–1144.

78. Kim S-H, Ha K-I, Cho Y-B, Ryu B-D, Oh I. Arthroscopic anterior stabilization of the shoulder. *J Bone Joint Surg.* 2003;85A:1511–1518.

79. Miller SL, Gothelf T, Hazrati Y, Gladstone JL, Cornwall Flatow EL, et al. Failed surgical management of partial thickness rotator cuff tears. *Orthopedics.* 2002;25:1255–1257.

80. Gardner E. The innervation of the elbow joint. *Anat Rec.* 1947;100:341–346.

81. Kaplan E. Treatment of tennis elbow (epicondylitis) by denervation. *J Bone Joint Surg.* 1959;41A:147–151.

82. Wilhelm A. Tennis elbow treatment of resistant cases by denervation. *J Bone Joint Surg.* 1996;21B:523–533.

83. DeJesus RA, Ducic I, Dellon AL. Denervation of the lateral humeral epicondyle for treatment of "failed tennis elbow." Paper presented at the American Association for Hand Surgery meeting, Palm Springs, CA, January 2004.

84. Dellon AL, Ducic I, DeJesus R. Medial humeral epicondylitis: neural origin of the medial epicondylitis? *J Reconstr Microsurg.* 2004;20:347.

85. Dellon AL. Partial Joint Denervation: First Applications to the Ankle, Shoulder, Elbow, and Hip. Plastic Surgery Educational Foundation Award presentation at American Society for Plastic Surgery meeting, Philadelphia, March 2004.

86. Dellon AL, Maloney CT Jr. Denervation of the temporomandibular nerve. In: *New Techniques in Plastic Surgery.* Siemionow M, editor. London: Springer Verlag, 2005.

87. Wilhelm A, Gieseler H. Die Behandlung der Epicondylitis humeri radialis durch Denervation [German]. *Chirurg.* 1962;33:118.

88. Rader A. Results of tibial nerve decompression in diabetics in terms of pain relief and recovery of sensibility. *J Amer Pod Med Assoc.* 2005:446–451.

6

Minimally Invasive and Endoscopic Techniques in Peripheral Nerve Surgery of the Hand and Forearm

Reimer Hoffmann

Introduction

Minimally invasive and endoscopic techniques are not new in surgery; in fact, they are well established in many fields, such as general and gynecological surgery. In hand surgery, only the endoscopic operation of the carpal tunnel syndrome has become an established technique.[1,2] In spite of an initial enthusiastic reception by many hand surgeons, this operation has not marked the beginning of a new "endoscopic" era in hand surgery. A high complication rate and the fact that it is technically demanding and relatively expensive are some of the reasons enthusiasm waned. An alternative for many hand surgeons became minimizing the incision for the open operation, to a point where the size of the incision was not larger than the one needed for the introduction of an endoscope.[3,4] This minimally invasive technique, however, has become popular only for carpal tunnel release.

Hand surgeons continue to look for broader applications for both minimally invasive and endoscopic surgery. It remains a challenge, therefore, to introduce minimally invasive and endoscopic techniques to hand surgery in a way that allows them to become a routine and useful aspect of this specialty. In this chapter we describe some of the techniques we have used to treat carpal tunnel syndrome, pronator syndrome, anterior interosseus syndrome, cubital tunnel syndrome, tennis elbow (including the posterior interosseus nerve), and the radial sensory nerve.

Endoscopic and Minimally Invasive Hand Surgery

Endoscopic surgery and minimally invasive surgery are not surgical techniques; rather, they are a completely new approach to surgery that enables us to see and to do more through much smaller incisions. The skin incision should follow the natural skin creases and, in most cases, will be transverse or oblique. The resulting scars are wonderfully inconspicuous. If possible, the incision should be at a distance from the area to be dissected to keep the internal and external scars separate.

As with other forms of endoscopic surgery, the surgeon needs to create a space to work in. Because we cannot inflate the soft tissue of an extremity with gas, as is done in abdominal surgery, we must create a space using a tunneling forceps of the appropriate size (Figure 6-1). With the blades of this forceps, the tissue layers we want to dissect can be gently separated.

For good visualization, we use specula and endoscopes attached to a light source. The specula are similar to those used in ENT surgery (Figure 6-1), and the endoscopes—originally designed for endoscopic face lifting—have dissectors of varying size and shape at their tip (Figure 6-1). With the specula, the tunnel can be opened in three directions, and with the endoscope, the soft tissue envelope can be held up, enabling the surgeon to introduce instruments and to dissect within this space.

When using illuminated specula, dissection is done under direct vision in the tunnel;

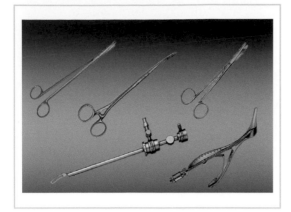

Figure 6-1. Instruments for endoscopic nerve decompression: tunneling forces (top middle), speculum (bottom right), endoscope with dissector on tip (bottom left).

when working with the endoscopes, dissection is observed and controlled on the monitor. The aim of endoscopic and minimally invasive surgery is to further enhance atraumatic technique.

Any surgical interference with tissue will invariably produce a scar. The less dissection through tissue layers that glide against one another, the less scarring we will get, and the more function will be preserved. Scarring is not only an aesthetic problem but may lead to tethering of tendons, nerves, and other structures. It impairs motion and can create pain. Tissue that is not cut but only spread will recover its natural functions much more quickly. When scarring is limited, tissues glide early when motion begins, and pain is less. Perioperative morbidity will be reduced and functional recovery will be faster. Therefore, patients can be encouraged to move early, and they will do so because they experience less pain. Therefore, time away from work is less and normal activities can be resumed early.

Arthroscopy has also shown that "less can be more." Although skin incisions are tiny when performing arthroscopy, the surgeon has a much better view of all joint compartments and can usually gain access to structures that are inaccessible during open surgery. With endoscopic and minimally invasive surgery of soft tissues, the same advantages are encountered. With the speculum and endoscope, we can often advance much further into our surgical field along the anatomical course when releasing a compressed nerve, without extending the skin incision. Therefore, it is quite possible that anomalous

fibrous bands that cross and compress a nerve are more often found and split than in a conventional procedure. This ability may contribute to a more radical nerve release and better results. Moreover, when operating with the endoscope, more magnification is possible—magnification comparable to a microscope—which further enhances the precision and completeness of dissection.

Endoscopic and minimally invasive techniques are not intended to replace standard techniques in hand and peripheral nerve surgery but to enhance and supplement them. Thus, these techniques are not for beginners but for surgeons who have already mastered the common techniques. This circumstance, however, as in other surgical specialties, will most likely change with time.

We are at the beginning of this era, and therefore new applications must be carefully explored and must also stand the test of time. In cooperation with instrument makers and endoscope manufacturers, new instruments must be designed to simplify and improve these new techniques.

In the following sections, we describe some techniques that we have successfully incorporated into my daily routine. Other techniques are still being refined. We have not addressed wrist arthroscopy here because it is a well established technique.

Carpal Tunnel Syndrome

Carpal tunnel syndrome is the most frequent nerve compression syndrome in every hand surgery practice.

The aim of surgery is the complete decompression of the median nerve by dividing the flexor retinaculum and the adjacent forearm fascia. Anyone turning to *Green's Operative Hand Surgery*[5] for advice and who follows the author's preferred method will be told to do a "classic open carpal tunnel release." (Figure 6-2) The author does not explain why this release is "classic," however. "Classic" in this context often means "historic." Although the open method certainly is justifiably safe for carpal tunnel release, particularly for the beginner, the incision shown in the book should be historical, in the sense that it is obsolete. An incision extending to the forearm must be strictly avoided—the only exception is a very proliferative tenosynovitis in

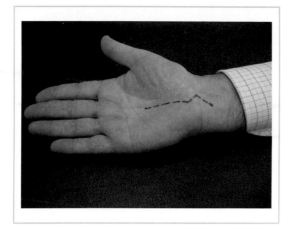

Figure 6-2. Incision for the "author's preferred method," as described in Green's hand surgery textbook.[5]

a rheumatoid patient—because a scar in this area often becomes hypertrophic and may cause social problems for the patient as it mimics the scar created in a suicide attempt.

The larger the incision in the palm, the greater the risk of cutting small cutaneous nerves in this area, which may subsequently lead to a painful scar secondary to small neuromata. A considerable number of patients experience pillar pain in the proximal palm near the wrist crease, pain that can be a postoperative problem, sometimes for many months. A scar in this area contributes to this problem.

Endoscopic technique should not be the surgeon's first choice for 2 reasons. First, endoscopic instruments are expensive, and because hand surgeons sometimes do several of these operations on one day, the surgery center would need quite a few instruments. Second, the technique is not safe enough. It may be so in expert hands, but carpal tunnel release is done by many surgeons without specialized training in hand surgery. The complications reported in the literature and encountered even by specialized hand surgeons are simply too high. This technique carries a risk because the anatomical structures cannot be visualized at all times during the procedure: there is a "blind" element involved.

We are using a minimally invasive technique with a short incision in the palm.[4] This technique, which requires very few instruments and a speculum for the "endoscopic" part, is easy to learn. The operation is performed with the patient under an either brachial plexus block or local anesthesia. A tourniquet to obtain a bloodless field is essential.

The principle is to operate from distal to proximal. The incision follows the longitudinal crease between the thenar and hypothenar eminence (Figure 6-3) and can be between 18 mm and 25 mm long. It lies over the distal third of the carpal tunnel. The subcutaneous tissue is separated down to the palmar aponeurosis. The fascia is divided, and its edges are retracted with 2-pronged skin hooks. The flexor retinaculum is exposed, and its distal part divided. The median nerve and its motor branch are identified. Whenever atypical musculature is found, at this or any other point in the carpal tunnel, an atypical motor branch variation must strongly be suspected. All anatomical variations[6] of the motor branch must be kept in mind to keep the procedure safe.

The deep transverse carpal ligament is cut with a 15 blade for 10 mm to 15 mm in a proximal direction, further exposing the median nerve. Before the final release, a tunnel is created using a needle holder as tunneling forceps, spreading the tissue between the palmar aponeurosis and the proximal part of the flexor retinaculum and the forearm fascia (Figure 6-4a). A speculum with a blade length of 50 mm is inserted into the tunnel and gently opened (Figure 6-4b). The inside of the tunnel is visualized, either by a light source attached to the speculum or by an external light. An excellent "endoscopic" view down the undivided part of the flexor retinaculum and the forearm fascia is obtained (Figure 6-5a).

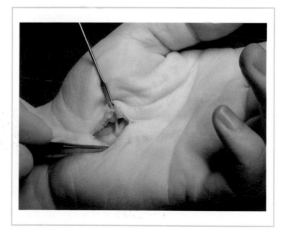

Figure 6-3. Small incision for minimally invasive, open carpal tunnel surgery. The motor branch of the median nerve has been dissected.

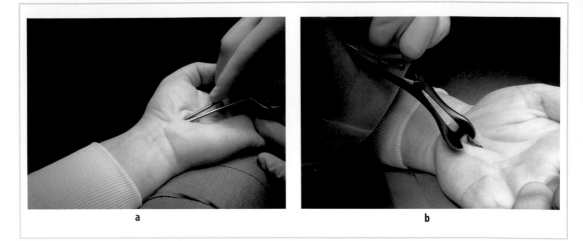

Figure 6-4. **a**) Tunneling with the needle holder (see text). **b**) Speculum inserted for viewing the undivided part of the flexor retinaculum and forearm fascia.

Retinaculum and fascia, kept taut with the speculum, are divided with the scalpel or, rarely, with scissors. The fascia is divided up to 3 cm proximal to the wrist crease (Figure 6-5b). Tenosynovectomy is possible without enlarging the skin incision. The only indications to open the skin incision down to the wrist crease are in rheumatoid or dialysis patients in whom large amounts of proliferative synovitis or amyloid tissue need to be excised.

Hemostasis is achieved with bipolar coagulation; a drain is rarely necessary. A bulky dressing is applied. We prefer to immobilize the wrist for a week in a dorsal splint. With some routine, this operation takes about 10 minutes from skin incision to finishing the dressing.

The technique combines the advantage of low morbidity of the endoscopic approach with the greater safety of the open method. Using a small, standard set of ordinary hand surgery instruments makes surgery very cost-effective ("safer-faster-cheaper"). We have used this method in more than 4000 patients and recommend it without any hesitation.

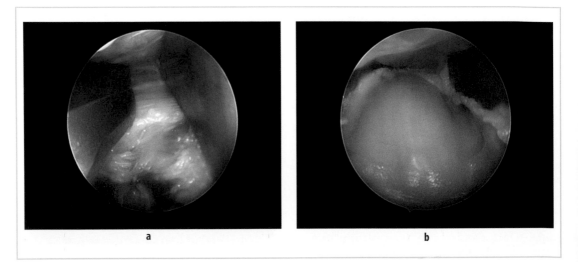

Figure 6-5. "Endoscopic" view with speculum. **a**) The undivided part of the flexor retinaculum and forearm fascia are clearly visible, as are the blades of the speculum. **b**) The flexor and adjacent forearm fascia completely divided.

Pronator Syndrome

Proximal median nerve compression is much less common than carpal tunnel syndrome, and it may be overlooked because the associated symptoms and physical signs may be vague.

Pronator syndrome resembles carpal tunnel syndrome in that numbness occurs in the same digits, weakness may develop in the thenar muscles, and pain is reported in the wrist and forearm. Paresthesia of the median-innervated fingers without physical signs of carpal tunnel or chronic pain in the proximal palmar region of the forearm resistant to conservative treatment should be considered to be the result of compression of the median nerve in the pronator tunnel. The potential sites of compression, however, are not only in the pronator muscle; therefore, it would be more adequate to term this condition "proximal median nerve compression."

The most proximal potential structure that can compress the median nerve the ligament of Struthers. This fibrous band runs from a supracondyloid process to the medial epicondyle, and the median nerve passes beneath it. Although the supracondyloid process is found in only 3% of patients, the ligament of Struthers is potentially present in everyone; thus, the proximal median nerve should be explored proximal to the elbow to be sure the nerve is not compressed at this level.

The next structure that can compress the median nerve is the lacertus fibrosus. The median nerve then passes through the pronator tunnel, which is formed by the two heads of the pronator teres, with their tendinous origins and fibrous edges. In addition, other fibrous bands may constrict the nerve as it passes through this muscle.

Distal to the pronator, the nerve passes through a tendinous arc formed by the origin of the flexor digitorum superficialis (FDS).[7] When decompressing the nerve, it is wise to follow the aforementioned course and not to leave any of the compression sites unreleased. Therefore, in the past[7] and still today, long incisions, from 12 cm to 20 cm, have been suggested.[5]

As in carpal tunnel syndrome, the aim of surgery in pronator syndrome is the complete decompression of the median nerve. All offending tendinous and fibrous structures crossing

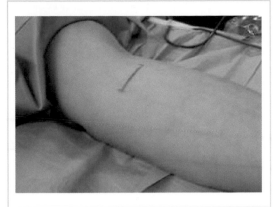

Figure 6-6. Skin incision for a minimally invasive approach to pronator tunnel release.

the median nerve must be released. The fleshy parts of the muscles involved are never "offending" structures and can be left intact. This circumstance makes the surgery less "offensive" and opens the door for a minimally invasive and endoscopic approach.

Following guidelines for safe endoscopic surgery, we expose the median nerve through a 3-to-4-cm transverse incision 2 cm to 3 cm distal from the cubital crease, on the ulnar-palmar aspect of the forearm (Figure 6-6). The fascia is exposed between the flexor carpi radialis and pronator teres. The median nerve can be easily located here by palpation (Figure 6-7a). The fascia is opened, and the muscle bellies are retracted radially and ulnarly with appropriately sized Langenbeck retractors (blade 3 cm wide and 5 cm to 6 cm long). A self-retaining retractor may be helpful distracting the wound margins in the distal-proximal direction. The nerve is dissected with ease under direct vision as far as possible (Figure 6-7b).

A subcutaneous tunnel is created distally and proximally. A 9-to-11-cm speculum is introduced, and forearm fascia and muscle raphe are transected first in a proximal direction. The endoscope is introduced, and dissection carried out as described for the surgery of cubital tunnel syndrome. The fibrous arcades and other constricting bands within the pronator and proximal to it are divided, and the nerve is completely decompressed up to 8 cm proximal to the cubital crease (Figure 6-8). The muscles themselves are left intact. The same procedure is done in a distal

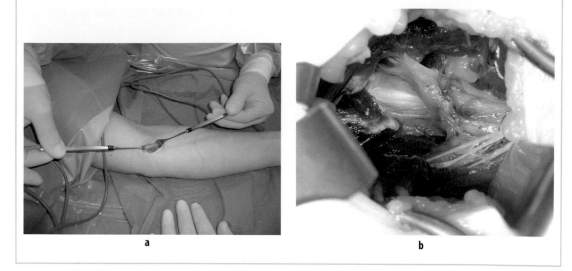

Figure 6-7. **a**) Exposure of the forearm fascia in a direct approach to dissecting the median nerve. **b**) Further direct dissection of the median nerve (left = distal). The muscular nerve branches, and first fibrous arcade are distal to the nerve.

direction. All branches of the nerve can be visualized, identified, and protected.

Fibrous arcades in the pronator tunnel are divided (Figures 6-9a and 6-9b). The anterior interosseus nerve can be followed and is completely decompressed (Figure 6-10). At the end of the endoscopic route, the FDS arc is located and divided (Figure 6-11). A suction drain is inserted and the wound closed. A bulky dressing is applied, and the upper arm is cast in plaster of Paris for 2 days. Postoperatively, patients are encouraged to move the arm, which is protected only by an elastic bandage.

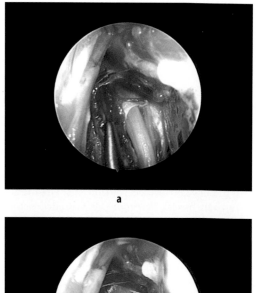

a

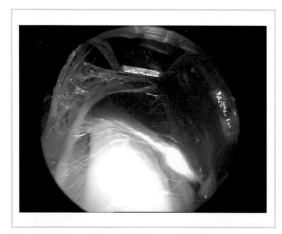

Figure 6-8. Endoscopic view of the fibrous arcade in the proximal pronator tunnel.

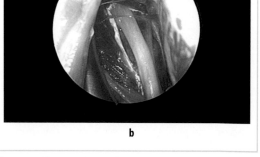

b

Figure 6-9. Fibrous arcade in the distal part of pronator tunnel **a**) before and **b**) after endoscopic release.

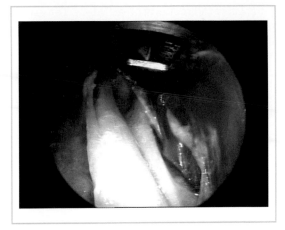

Figure 6-10. Endoscopic view of the anterior interosseus nerve branching off median nerve and crossing under the tendinous edge (right).

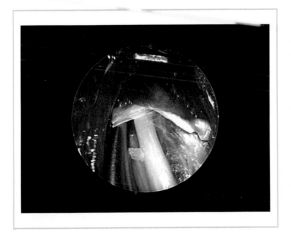

Figure 6-11. Endoscopic view of the flexor digitorum superficialis arc before division.

We can only report preliminary results in 5 patients, but they are very encouraging. All patients were successfully relieved of their symptoms and had full range of elbow motion within 5 to 6 days. The least we can say at this early stage is that the results of endoscopic management of this nerve entrapment are equal to the open method but that morbidity is much less and early rehabilitation much faster.

Anterior Interosseus Syndrome

Clinically, the anterior interosseus syndrome is much more obvious and easier to diagnose than the pronator syndrome.[7] Patients present with weakness or palsy of the muscles innervated by the anterior interosseus nerve, the flexor pollicis longus, the flexor digitorum profundus to the index finger, and the pronator quadratus. In contrast to pronator syndrome, electromyography of the FPL is usually helpful to confirm the diagnosis. Anterior interosseus palsy may be caused by a neuritis (Parsonage-Turner syndrome), which must be ruled out by a neurologist before surgery.

Although clinical findings usually identify the site of compression, fascicular compression within the median nerve may confound the location.[8] Although we do not perform an internal neurolysis in all cases of anterior interosseus syndrome, we completely decompress the median nerve as described for pronator syndrome, in addition to a meticulous decompression of the anterior interosseus nerve and all its branches.

The minimally invasive and endoscopic approach, naturally, is similar to that in the pronator syndrome. We routinely identify the level where the anterior interosseus branches off the median nerve stem by neuroultrasound preoperatively so that the skin incision can be placed more precisely. The anterior interosseus branch is identified and followed to its muscular branches, especially the one innervating the flexor pollicis, to make sure every potential compression is addressed. At this stage of our endoscopic experience, we believe this dissection should be done under direct vision. Once all constricting elements have been released, the median nerve is endoscopically decompressed as described above.

Cubital Tunnel Syndrome

The overall success rate of the different surgical procedures for cubital tunnel syndrome, which is the second most frequent nerve entrapment of the arm, is between 80% and 90%.[5] Still, the debate on in situ ("simple") nerve decompression versus anterior transposition continues.[9,10,11] If in situ decompression gives the same good success rate,[12,13] one would think that a complex procedure, such as the anterior transposition of the ulnar nerve, especially its most aggressive submuscular version, would have no place. Why would a surgeon unnecessarily risk potential complications, such as devascularization of the nerve, painful extension of elbow, a new compression site by kinking, and perineural fibrosis? These are only a few examples of potential complications of anterior transposition.

A surgeon seeking advice from *Green's Operative Hand Surgery* will be told that the indications for in situ decompression are "mild or intermittent symptoms in a nonsubluxating ulnar nerve when there is normal osseous anatomy, absence of pain around the medial epicondyle, and findings are consistent with compression under the fibrous arcade." The surgeon will then be advised to do a limited in situ decompression, extending down to 5 cm distal from the medial epicondyle. Alternatively, a subcutaneous anterior transposition will be recommended for patients "with bony deformity or subluxation or dislocation of the nerve or for severe cases with motor involvement." The recommended technique involves a 15-cm skin incision and extensive dissection, up to 8 cm proximally and at least 7 cm distally. How these recommendations fit with the overall statement that any technique will give good results must be very confusing for the reader.

We believe that there are true elements in both procedures. Open in situ decompression is safe, but it may not be extensive enough in all cases. The extensive dissection and decompression necessary for a nerve transposition are effective, but they are also laden with many risks and dangers.

The endoscopic approach is not new. Tsu-Min Tsai et al.[14] used an endoscopic technique for cubital tunnel syndrome as early as 1992. They concluded that their results were no better than those of other standard techniques. The description of their technique has some analogy to the techniques used for endoscopic surgery for carpal tunnel syndrome. They describe the extensive division of the forearm fascia only.

Our endoscopic operation for cubital tunnel syndrome is a "long-distance" in situ decompression. We combine the advantages of both procedures and minimize the risks.

We apply the same general principles for minimal invasive and endoscopic surgery as outlined above: exposing the nerve through a small incision, creating space with a tunneling forceps along the course of the ulnar nerve, and visualization with speculum and endoscope.

The operation is performed with the patient under plexus block or general anesthesia. A pneumatic tourniquet is always used. Draping must allow full mobility of the elbow. The arm is positioned in 90° abduction on a standard hand table, and the surgeon flexes and supinates the arm to face the cubital tunnel area.

The ulnar nerve is palpated, and a 15-to-25-mm incision is made in the retrocondylar groove along the natural skin creases, usually in an oblique fashion. The dissection is carried down to the tunnel roof, which is opened. Clearly recognizable by its vasa nervorum, the nerve is identified (Figure 6-12). A tunneling forceps is introduced distally and proximally into the space between the fascia and subcutaneous tissue. By spreading the blunt-tipped forceps, a generous space is created, which permits the insertion of instruments (Figure 6-13). Spreading of the instrument must not be forceful to avoid stretching the cutaneous nerves in this area, especially the ulnar antebrachial cutaneous nerve.

First, an illuminated speculum (blade length 9-to-11 cm) is inserted (Figure 6-14a), and Osborne's ligament (sometimes called the "cubital tunnel retinaculum") is divided under direct vision (Figure 6-14b,c). With the use of the speculum alone, the fascial tunnel roof can be incised up to 5 cm distally and proximally from the epicondyle (Figure 6-14d).

A 4-mm, 30° endoscope with a blunt dissector on its tip (STORZ Inc.) is introduced and slowly advanced distally (Figure 6-15). Lifting up the soft tissue envelope of the forearm with the dissector creates a generous space to view the nerve and its surrounding anatomy. All dissection and cutting is done with blunt-tipped scissors

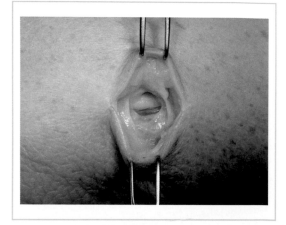

Figure 6-12. Retrocondylar dissection of the ulnar nerve through a small incision. The nerve is always identifiable by the vasa nervorum.

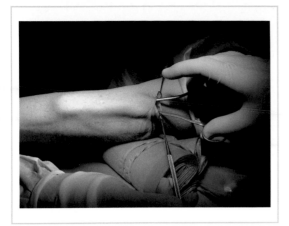

Figure 6-13. Distal tunneling of the cubital tunnel (see text).

between 17cm and 23cm long. Under monitor vision, the forearm fascia is divided to a point 10cm to 14cm distally from the epicondyle (Figure 6-16). Care must be taken not to injure the cutaneous nerve branches or the veins that may cross the fascia. Once the fascia has been divided, the endoscope is carefully pulled back, and further dissection is carried out close to the nerve.

The next step is to divide the two muscular heads of the flexor carpi ulnaris and to release of all fibrous bands crossing the nerve. Distally from Osborne's ligament, the fascia between the two heads of the flexor carpi ulnaris (FCU) is

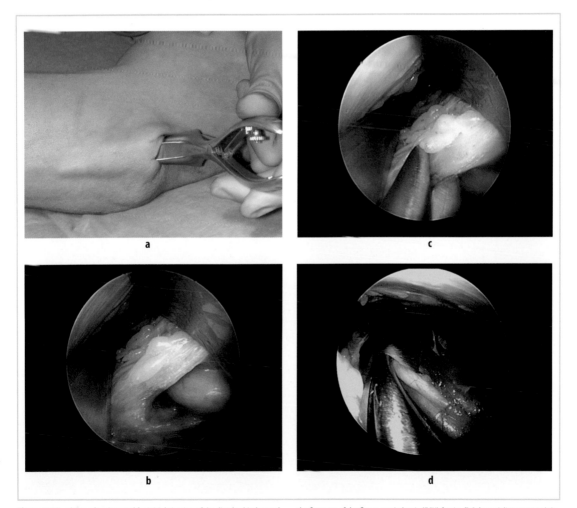

Figure 6-14. **a**) Speculum inserted for initial viewing of the distal cubital tunnel. **b**) Ulnar nerve entering the cubital tunnel under Osborne's ligament (cubital retinaculum). **c**) Speculum view of scissors about to cut Osborne's ligament and the first part of the flexor carpi ulnaris (FCU) fascia. **d**) Osborne's ligament and the first part of the FCU fascia released. The scissors blades are under the first fibrous arcade between the two heads of the FCU.

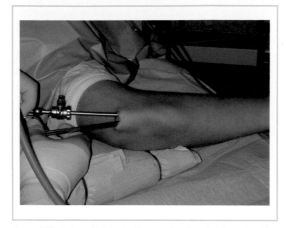

Figure 6-15. Endoscopic dissection 10 cm to 12 cm from the ulnar epicondyle.

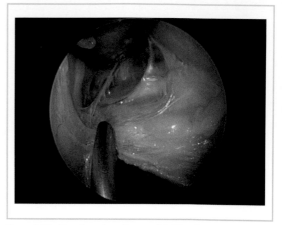

Figure 6-16. Dissecting scissors "en route," dividing the superficial forearm fascia 8 cm to 10 cm from the retro-condylar groove. A tiny nerve, identifiable by the vasa nervorum, crosses fascia distal from the scissors.

divided. About 3 cm distal from the medial epicondyle, the first fibrous arcade can be located and divided. Then the raphe between the two muscular elements of the FCU is transected, and all constricting elements up to a distance of perhaps 12 cm (measured from the middle of the retrocondylar groove) are divided. In the course of this dissection, all muscle branches can be seen and protected (Figure 6-17). We have regularly observed and divided distinct fibrous arcades at 5 cm, 7 cm, and 9 cm from the epicondyle (Figure 6-18). Only rarely is it necessary to

clip or cauterize a vessel. Lax adipose soft tissue of the forearm, as sometimes seen in elderly women, makes the dissection difficult, mainly because the optic needs repeated cleaning and some loose fatty tissue must be removed.

Proximally, the tunnel roof is decompressed in the same fashion. The fascia, but not the intermuscular septum, is divided 8 cm to 10 cm from the retrocondylar groove. No constricting elements have been observed in this area. A CH 8 suction drain may be inserted, and a bulky dressing applied. Then the tourniquet is

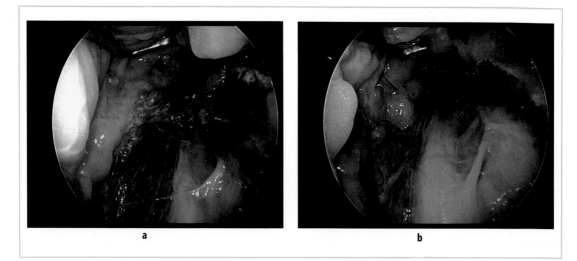

a

b

Figure 6-17. Magnified endoscopic view of nerve branches in the cubital tunnel.

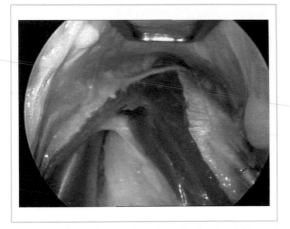

Figure 6-18. The 3rd fibrous arcade at the distal end of the cubital tunnel about 9 cm from the retro-condylar groove. The two layers of dissection are shown: the superficial fascia already split, and the arcade close to the nerve before release.

loosened. Patients are allowed to move their elbow but are instructed to avoid resting the arm in flexion for 4 to 6 weeks, to prevent secondary nerve subluxation. After 3 days, an elastic elbow bandage is prescribed for 4 to 6 weeks.

To validate the need for an extensive distal release of the ulnar nerve in patients with cubital tunnel syndrome, we evaluated the ulnar nerve anatomy in its distal course in the forearm between the two heads of the FCU.

All cadaver specimens studied showed evidence of fascial bands crossing the ulnar nerve on its route between the two heads of the FCU. After the intermuscular septum between the two heads of the FCU were dissected, three distinct zones of fascial thickening, seen as visible bands, were encountered (Figure 6-19a). The first band was seen 3 cm from the middle of the retrocondylar groove, and it was 1.5 cm wide, ending 4.5 cm from the middle of the groove. The second band originated 5 cm distal to the middle of the groove and was narrower, measuring only 0.5 cm in width. It ended 5.5 cm distal from the groove. The third band originated 7 cm distal from the groove. This band was the most prominent and measured 2 cm in width. This band extended up to 9 cm from the middle of the groove (Figure 6-19b).

The results from this procedure are encouraging. Between March 2001 and February 2005, about 150 patients underwent this procedure, of which 95% reported improvement of symptoms within 24 hours after surgery and continued to improve thereafter. There were no recurrences. Postoperative nerve subluxation did not occur. In the longer term, 93% of patients had excellent and good results; more than 90% had full elbow motion within 2 days after surgery and the rest, within a week.

In 75 patients, the following complications were found. Algodystrophy developed in 1 patient, and the result was poor. There were 4 cases of superficial hematoma. All resolved within a week, and no particular treatment was

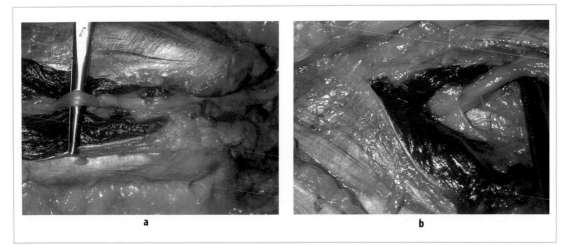

Figure 6-19. a) Cadaver dissection of the ulnar nerve in the cubital tunnel showing fibrous thickening around the nerve. **b)** "Anterior transposition" of the ulnar nerve demonstrating the possibility of a new nerve compression and kinking against the cut edge of the fascia and fibrous arcade.

necessary. In 9 patients, hypesthesia developed in the skin innervated by the ulnar antebrachial cutaneous nerve, most likely from stretching of the nerve during the tunneling procedure. In all but 1 patient, hypesthesia resolved within 3 months.

The advantages of our endoscopic technique for cubital tunnel syndrome are mainly its simplicity and low morbidity. The nerve is efficiently decompressed over a long distance in its own habitat. Lesions of cutaneous nerve branches are avoided because of the very small incision. The soft tissue envelope over the ulnar nerve remains intact and stabilizes the nerve. No scars impair the free gliding of the tissue layers.

Tennis Elbow (Including Radial Tunnel Syndrome)

The cause of chronic pain in the lateral elbow, somewhat misleadingly termed "tennis elbow," is still unknown, which may be why a variety of surgical procedures have been described to treat it, including denervation,[18] extensor tendon release,[15] and decompression of the posterior interosseus nerve (PIN).[16]

Surgery, in our opinion, is indicated if repeated attempts of nonoperative treatment have failed. Only in about 10% of our patients, where symptoms and physical signs suggest an isolated epicondylitis, do we limit surgery to the epicondylar area, denervating the lateral elbow and releasing all extensors originating from the lateral epicondyle. In all other cases, we combine this procedure with a decompression of the PIN. The reason for this combination is that most often the lateral epicondyle and the radial tunnel are equally tender. Both conditions seem inseparably connected to us and are almost indistinguishable by clinical examination. Electromyography is rarely helpful for patients with tennis elbow but may prove useful if a PIN palsy is present.

For many years, we have used standard incisions with little modification from those seen in most textbooks.[4,5] Scars from these incisions cause problems, not only aesthetically. The more extensive the incision, the higher the risk of severing one of the many cutaneous nerve branches in this area and to produce a painful neuroma. There is hardly any soft tissue padding on the epicondyle, so the scar may tether down to the bone, become painful, and impair motion. Moreover, to allow access to the radial tunnel, it must be fairly long, up to 10 cm or more.

Following our principles for minimally invasive and endoscopic techniques, we now perform the combined operation from a 4-cm incision over the radial tunnel (Figure 6-20), about 5 cm distal from the epicondyle. The incision is oblique or transverse, depending on the direction of the skin creases, which are easily detected by lightly squeezing the skin. When exposing the fascia, all cutaneous branches of the area must be protected. With the tunneling forceps, we create a space in the periepicondylar area (Figure 6-21). An illuminated speculum (blade length 9 to 11 cm) is inserted, giving a perfect view of the epicondyle and its surrounding structures (Figure 6-22a). Through the speculum, we continue with the epifascial detachment of the flaps, thereby severing tiny pain-transmitting branches of the dorsal cutaneous antebrachial nerve.

Another small nerve branch running with the radial intermuscular septum is cauterized about 3 cm proximal of the epicondyle. The next step is the complete release of all extensor tendon origins between epicondyle and radial head, leaving the joint capsule intact (Figure 6-22b). Excellent vision allows for meticulous hemostasis with a bipolar micro forceps.

The radial nerve is approached transmuscularly in its plane between the extensor digitorum and the extensor carpi radialis brevis.[7] If the

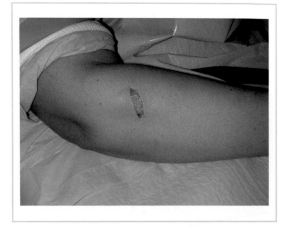

Figure 6-20. Incision, following the skin crease, for a minimally invasive approach to the peri-epicondylar area and radial tunnel of the posterior interosseus nerve.

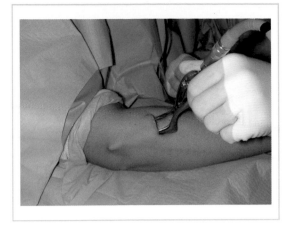

Figure 6-21. Insertion of the speculum (blade length, 11 cm) for viewing the peri-epicondylar area.

nerve is explored in connection with the procedure described above, we continue to separate the aponeurosis between the desoriginated muscles and develop the plane from there. If radial nerve decompression is done as a separate operation, it is easier to open the raphe between the extensor carpi radialis brevis and the extensor digitorum more distally.

After entering the intermuscular plane, dissection is usually blunt, and large Langenbecks are inserted to retract the brachioradialis muscle mass and the extensor muscles to either side, exposing the PIN. As a result of the very small incision, this part of the operation is tedious and difficult and requires experience with dissecting the anatomy around Frohse's arcade. It also requires excellent assistance because the retractors must be pulled fairly hard but, at the same time, no pressure is allowed on the nerve branches. Usually incising the tendinous margin of the extensor carpi radialis brevis greatly helps to expose the supinator muscle and Frohse's arcade at its proximal edge. We divide the arcade and all aponeurotic parts of the supinator, but not the fleshy part of the muscle. Sometimes vascular bundles crossing the PIN must be hemoclipped or cauterized.

We palpate carefully in a proximal direction along the radial nerve, under the brachioradialis, for more proximal compression sites. A suction drain may be inserted, and the wound is always closed in two layers, using intracutaneous skin closure. An upper arm dorsal splint is applied for 2 days. Afterwards, patients are instructed to move their elbow, which is protected by an elastic bandage. Physiotherapy is prescribed if necessary.

We have used this minimally invasive technique since February 2004 in about 20 patients. It is much too early to recommend it, especially for radial nerve decompression "through a keyhole" because it is technically quite demanding. We have been impressed, however, with the very low morbidity and good functional results. Patients regained full range of motion earlier than with our conventional method, which

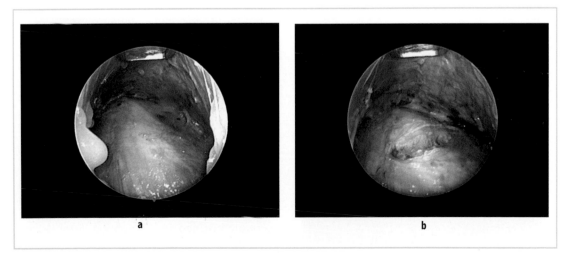

a   b

Figure 6-22. a) Endoscopic view of the peri-epicondylar area. The lateral epicondyle and extensor tendon origins are visible. **b**) The peri-epicondylar area after release of the extensor tendon origins.

required immobilization for 8 to 12 days. All patients were delighted with the inconspicuous scar, especially those who had a larger longitudinal scar from a previous operation on the other elbow.

Radial Sensory Nerve Compression

Entrapment of the radial sensory nerve (RSN) at the mid forearm is certainly less frequent than the compression neuropathies mentioned above. Nevertheless, it is a cause of chronic pain and discomfort in the radial forearm. Many patients with this entrapment are referred with a diagnosis of de Quervain's tendovaginitis. They should be carefully examined to exclude the diagnosis of RSN compression. Both conditions can exist at the same time. The RSN is usually compressed between the tendinous edges of the extensor carpi radialis longus and the brachioradialis between the mid- and distal third of the radial forearm. The aim of surgery is to release the fascia between these muscles. Conventional surgery with a 6-cm skin incision is effective.[17]

Our 2-cm transverse incision is at the junction of the mid and distal third of the radial circumference of the forearm. The RSN is identified and dissected (Figure 6-23). Care must be taken not to injure any other cutaneous nerves in this area. The tunneling is done as described above, and the endoscope is gently introduced. Being so

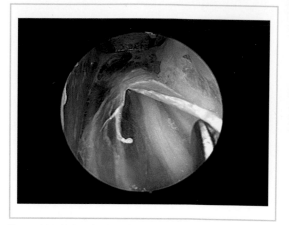

Figure 6-24. Endoscopic view of a partially divided fascia between the tendons of brachioradialis (right) and the extensor carpi radialis longus muscles (left).

close to the nerve and working through a very small incision, the endoscope must also be removed carefully to avoid injuring the nerve with the edges of the dissector. As the endoscope is moved forward and the dissection proceeds, the junction between the tendons of the brachioradialis and the extensor carpi radialis longus cannot be missed. The fascia between the tendons is incised, and the incision is carried further until the fleshy part of the muscles is reached (Figure 6-24). At the magnified sight of the sharp tendinous edge of the brachioradialis, one might be tempted to incise this tendon, which is not necessary and, in our opinion, would only create scarring.

When de Quervain's tendovaginitis requires surgery as well, it can be performed through the same incision. For this purpose, a smaller endoscope dissector is used. With the RSN as a guideline, the roof of the first extensor compartment, which is usually thickened, is found. A scalpel with a 15 blade and a long handle is introduced, and the compartment is incised. The compartment may be released with the scalpel or scissors. If an accessory compartment is present, this is dealt with similarly. The results are usually very good. No open surgical method for this condition leaves the delicate RSN so undisturbed as this endoscopic procedure. The extra trouble is therefore justified, in our opinion. After decompressing the RSN, with or without release of the first tendon compartment, we apply a thumb spica for 3 to 4 days.

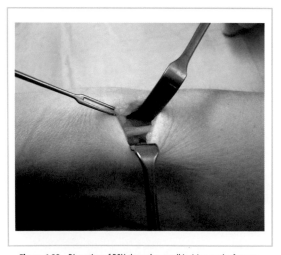

Figure 6-23. Dissection of RSN through a small incision on the forearm.

References

1. Agee JM, McCarroll HR, North ER. Endoscopic carpal tunnel release using the single proximal incision technique. *Hand Clin.* 1994;10:647–659.
2. Chow JC. Endoscopic release of the carpal ligament: a new technique for carpal tunnel syndrome. *Arthroscopy.* 1989;5:19–24.
3. Bromley GS. Minimal-incision open carpal tunnel decompression. *J Hand Surg.* 1994;19A:119–120.
4. Hoffmann R. *Checkliste Handchirurgie.* 2nd ed. Stuttgart: Thieme, 1999.
5. Szabo RM. Entrapment and compression neuropathies. In Green DP, Hotchkiss RN, Pederson WC, Editors. *Greens Operative Hand Surgery.* 4th ed. Philadelphia: Churchill Livingstone, 1999.
6. Lanz U. Anatomical variations of the median nerve in the carpal tunnel. *J Hand Surg.* 1977;2A:44–53.
7. Spinner M. *Injuries to the Major Branches of Peripheral Nerves of the Forearm.* Philadelphia: W.B. Saunders, 1978.
8. Nagano A, Shibata K, Tokimura H, Yamamoto S, Tajiri Y. Spontaneous anterior interosseus nerve palsy with hourglass-like fascicular constriction within the main trunk of the median nerve. *J Hand Surg.* 1996;21A: 266–270.
9. Heithoff SJ, Millender LH, Nalebuff EA, Petruska AJ jr. Medial epicondylectomy for the treatment of ulnar nerve compression at the elbow. *J Hand Surg.* 1990;15A:22–29.
10. Heithoff SJ. Cubital tunnel syndrome does not require transposition of the ulnar nerve. *J Hand Surg.* 1999;24A:898–905.
11. Kleinman WB, Bishop AT. Anterior intramuscular transposition of the ulnar nerve. *J Hand Surg.* 1989;14A:972–979.
12. Assmus H. The cubital tunnel syndrome with and without morphological alterations treated by simple decompression: results in 523 cases. *Nervenarzt.* 1994;65:846–853.
13. Nathan PA, Keniston RC, Meadows KD. Outcome study of ulnar nerve compression at the elbow treated with simple decompression and early programme of physical therapy. *J Hand Surg.* 1995;20B:628–637.
14. Tsai T, Chen I, Majd ME, Lim B. Cubital tunnel release with endoscopic assistance: results of a new technique. *J Hand Surg.* 1999;24A:21–29.
15. Hohmann G. Über den Tennisellenbogen. *Verhandlung der Deutschen orthopädischen Gesellschaft.* 1929;21: 349–354.
16. Lister GD, Belsole RB, Kleinert HE. The radial tunnel syndrome. *J Hand Surg.* 1979;4A:52–59.
17. Dellon AL, Mackinnon SE. Radial sensory nerve entrapment in the forearm. *J Hand Surg.* 1986;11A: 199–205.
18. Wilhelm A. Tennis elbow: treatment of resistant cases by denervation. *J Hand Surg* [Br]. 1996;21:523–533.

7

Soft Tissue Reconstruction with Perforator Flaps

Phillip N. Blondeel

Introduction

Perforator flaps have become increasingly popular among surgeons over recent years. They are an elegant solution to many reconstructive problems. For this reason, they are positioned near the top of the reconstructive ladder and are considered an elegant upgrade of musculocutaneous and fasciocutaneous flaps. Passive muscle and fascial carriers are no longer required to ensure flap vascularity, and, by virtue of their composition, perforator flaps permit excellent "like-for-like" tissue replacement with minimal aesthetic or functional donor morbidity. Perforator flaps are usually thin, pliable, easily moldable flaps that are well suited to resurfacing work. They are also ideal for reconstructing pliable organs, such as the tongue, or for molding to complex contours, as in head and neck surgery. Perforator flaps with large quantities of subcutaneous fat have proved ideal for reconstructing the breast.

A perforator flap is defined as a flap of skin and subcutaneous tissue, which is supplied by an isolated perforator vessel. Perforators pass from their source vessel to the skin surface, either through or between the deep tissues (mostly muscle). Any vessel that traverses through muscle before perforating the outer layer of the deep fascia to supply the overlying skin is termed a "myocutaneous perforator," and the resultant flap is called a "myocutaneous perforator flap." A vessel that traverses through a septum, that is, between the muscle bellies, is designated a "septocutaneous perforator" and the resultant flap is termed a "septocutaneous perforator flap."[1]

The Evolution of Perforator Flaps

The evolution of perforator flaps has been intimately related to a growing knowledge of the skin's blood supply and to the history of musculocutaneous and fasciocutaneous flap development. In 1889, Carl Manchot[2] published his seminal work on the arteries of the skin, marking the beginning of a rational understanding of flap viability. In 1936, this work was enhanced and expanded on by Michel Salmon's[3] studies using radio-opaque injection techniques. The research and clinical experience of Esser[4], Milton[5], Bakamjian[6], McGregor and Morgan[7], and a number of other pioneers led to the understanding that large subcutaneous vessels were necessary for large flaps to survive. The principles of the "axial" and "random" pattern flaps rapidly gained popularity.

Ian Taylor's[8] angiosome concept was a timely rediscovery and expansion of the work of Manchot and Salmon. Lead oxide injection studies of fresh cadavers revealed the existence of three-dimensional composite blocks of tissue (from bone to skin) supplied by a single source artery. The individual angiosomes varied in size, and each was linked to the next block of tissue or angiosome by anastomotic arteries. In total, 374 cutaneous perforators greater than 0.5 mm were mapped to the human body, each linked to the others by anastomotic, reduced-caliber "choke" arteries to form a continuous vascular network, most notably in the subdermal plexus. Current skin flap design is based on the concept of angiosomes; a viable flap can safely incorporate the angiosome supplied by the source artery and one adjacent anatomical cutaneous vascular territory.

The immediate precursor of the perforator flaps came in 1989, when Isao Koshima[9] published ground-breaking work on an inferior epigastric artery skin flap, without the rectus abdominis, that was pedicled on a single vessel that perforated the deep fascia and emanated from the deep inferior epigastric artery. The location and size of hitherto unrecognized vessels and the volume of tissue each vessel could sustain now warranted review and further study.

Taylor defines a cutaneous perforator as "any vessel that perforates the outer layer of the deep fascia to supply the overlying subcutaneous fat and skin."[10] The simplest way to define a perforator flap is based on the perforator vessels; thus Nakajima's direct and indirect perforators[11] nourish direct and indirect perforator flaps, respectively. The Gent consensus after the Fifth International Course on Perforator Flaps in 2001[1,12] sought to distinguish between musculocutaneous and septocutaneous perforator flaps. It was generally agreed that the intramuscular dissection required to dissect free the musculocutaneous (indirect) perforator was vastly different from that required to dissect a septocutaneous or direct perforator. Fu Chan Wei[13] argues that a true perforator is a cutaneous vessel that penetrates muscle, in addition to piercing the fascia to reach the skin. He derives the word "perforator" from the Latin *perforare*, meaning "to bore through," and supports the view that direct cutaneous vessels or those passing between muscles (septocutaneous) require simpler dissection techniques and thus do not represent "true" perforator flaps.

The "true" perforator or myocutaneous flaps are now named according to the source vessel. However, several different myocutaneous perforator flaps may be derived from a single source vessel. In these cases, the muscle through which the perforator passes is abbreviated and italicized to indicate the anatomic origin of the flap.

Thus, LCFAP-*vl* refers to the myocutaneous perforator derived from the lateral circumflex femoral artery and perforating the vastus lateralis; that is, the anterolateral thigh flap (ALT). The standardized nomenclature is rather cumbersome and is perhaps more useful as a retrospective tool; popular names, such as "ALT flap," are still in common use.

Perforator Flap Surgery

The success of all surgical procedures—especially perforator flap surgery—lies in the planning. After evaluating the location and dimensions of the defect and the general condition of the patient, an appropriate perforator flap should be selected. Perforator flaps may be raised either pedicled or free, and due consideration should be given to theater logistics and adequate peri and post-operative monitoring.

Preoperative investigative tools may include color Duplex scanning, an operator-dependent but useful way of visualizing the perforator vessels beforehand. Duplex scanning can assess the number, location, and size of perforators and also estimate the flow through the vessels.

Duplex scanning is more effective for some perforator flaps than others.[14] Alternatively, a simple hand-held 5-MHz to 8-MHz Doppler flow meter can locate audible perforators. Examining the donor area for scarring, tissue volume and quality, and local skin laxity is invaluable.

Dissecting the perforator flap itself is meticulous and requires a bloodless field, wide exposure of the vessels, loupe magnification, and careful ligation of all side branches of the vessels (Figure 7-1). The pedicle is freed by splitting the muscle fibres along the line of the muscle, to reduce muscle damage and subsequent functional deficit. Nerves should also be preserved. Postoperative care is the same as that for other free flaps.

The main advantage of perforator flaps is their low donor site morbidity. The majority of

Figure 7-1. a,b) Preoperative pictures of a middle-aged woman with invasive ductular breast carcinoma of the left breast, immediately after open biopsy through a supra-areolar scar. **c)** Intraoperative picture (right = cranial; left = caudal) of the dissection of a lateral perforator of the left rectus abdominis muscle between the umbilicus and the pubis. The fat of the flap, seen in the top of the picture, is folded medially; the deep (rectus) fascia (bottom of the picture) and muscle are split; and the deep inferior epigastric vessels are dissected from in between. The perforator has been isolated (white arrow), as well as the medial and lateral branches of the motor nerves (black arrows). Wide exposure and a bloodless field are the keys to success. **d,e)** Postoperative images after skin-sparing mastectomy, immediate autologous breast reconstruction with a DIEAP flap, nipple reconstruction, and areolar tattooing.

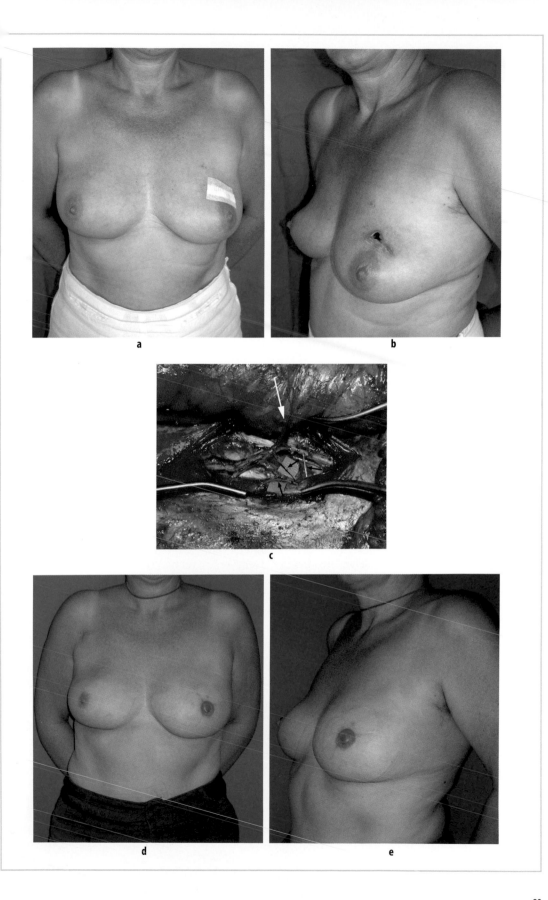

a

b

c

d

e

donor sites are designed to be closed directly, and the underlying muscle and its nerve supply are preserved; therefore, there is no functional deficit and no requirement for mesh closure.

By virtue of being muscle-sparing, the perforator flap itself is thin and pliable, composed of only skin, subcutaneous tissue and perhaps fascia. The vascular integrity of the flap is ensured as long as the angiosome principle is adhered to; therefore, the flaps may be as large or as small as required. Because no muscle is taken with the flap, it is not prone to atrophy or muscle fibrosis that might lead to shrinkage or distortion with time. Perforator flaps may be made sensate if harvested with their nerve supply.[15] The vascular pedicle can be made as long or as short as required, the diameter of the perforator rarely being an issue. Evidence also suggests faster recovery with perforator flaps, leading to shorter hospital stays[16], less analgesia[17], and more cost-effective care.[16]

The disadvantages of perforator flaps are largely related to the learning curve. Initially, dissection takes longer, leading to extended operating times in the beginning of the learning curve. The standard plastic surgery techniques of meticulous dissection, bloodless field, and so on, have to be rigorously applied. The perforator vessels may be small and prone to spasm. They are, however, relatively robust. The worst insult that can be applied to any perforator flap is traction or avulsion of the perforators during the dissection as they enter the flap.

Perforator flaps lend themselves to being used as either pedicled or free flaps. They are ideal "like-for-like" tissue replacements in tissue resurfacing work because often only skin and soft tissue are resected or lost. The pliable flaps are excellent for the difficult contour resurfacing associated with much head and neck surgery. Organs suited to reconstruction with thin perforator flaps include the perineum, vagina, tongue, and penis; alternatively, the bulky perforator flaps (DIEAP and S-GAP) are ideally suited for reconstructing the breast. Perforator flaps also lend themselves to pediatric use because they maintain the growing potential of the child. The perforator vessels are proportionally larger, and again, donor site morbidity is minimal.

As a separate perforator flap can be designed on any single perforator vessel, at least 374 perforator flaps can be described.

Types of Perforator Flaps

One of the first and most popular of all perforator flaps is the deep inferior epigastric artery perforator (DIEAP) flap. Its usefulness arises from the large area of lower abdominal tissue that can be sustained on a single perforator and the fact that the underlying subcutaneous tissue is thick. The resultant large, soft, bulky flap composed of skin and subcutaneous fat is an ideal "like-for-like" match for breast reconstruction (Figure 7-1).[18,19]

The ensuing flap, composed of only skin and fat, approximates the shape, texture, and movement of the breast. The color match is usually adequate. In a subcutaneous or skin-sparing mastectomy, the skin envelope of the original breast is preserved and the DIEAP flap is de-epithelialized and buried.

Koshima[20] presented a variant of the DIEAP flap that he named the "paraumbilical perforator" (PUP) flap. Pedicle dissection was limited to the perforator vessels superficial to the anterior rectus sheath; thus, donor morbidity was minimized by preserving the integrity of the anterior rectus sheath. The flap was rapidly and easily harvested, obviously at the expense of pedicle length and caliber. The flap was applied mainly to repair superficial defects with superficial recipient vessels[21] or as a de-epithelialized flap under subcutaneous cover.[22]

Donor functional morbidity has been studied intensively and compared directly against the transverse rectus abdominis myocutaneous (TRAM) flap. The advantages of the DIEAP over the TRAM flap in abdominal wall strength have been described,[23] in both retrospective[24] and prospective[25] studies; in addition, the costs and benefits[16] and the reduction in post-operative pain[17] have been identified.

The superior gluteal artery perforator (S-GAP) flap, first described by Koshima[26] for repairing sacral pressure sores, is another useful and increasingly widely used perforator flap. The S-GAP flap has become the flap of second choice for breast reconstruction. The flap is composed of skin and the thick subcutaneous fat of the buttock. Being more rigid, the gluteal fat provides greater projection than does the DIEAP for the smaller volume of flap. The S-GAP can also be re-innervated to allow sensate breast reconstruction.[15] Again, donor morbidity is minimal, the scar is hidden by most underwear, gluteus maximus muscle and function is retained, and the sciatic nerve is not exposed, which avoids accidental damage during surgery. In some care units, the pedicled S-GAP has become the flap of first choice in managing sacral pressure sores. The S-GAP tissue adequately replaces local soft tissue loss, without sacrificing future local reconstructive options, such as a myocutaneous flap.

Since it was first described in 1984,[27] the anterolateral thigh (ALT) flap has come to be described as the "ideal soft-tissue flap." This title reflects the versatility of the large, pliable flap that is harvested from the anterolateral thigh and the resultant minimal donor morbidity. The skin is vascularized by either muscular or septal perforators that originate in the descending branch of the lateral circumflex femoris artery and variably pierce the vastus lateralis muscle (LCFAP-*vl* flap).

The ALT flap has largely taken over the role of the free radial forearm flap in head and neck reconstruction. The ALT is supplied by a perforator from the descending branch of the lateral circumflex femoral artery and does not require the sacrifice of a major vessel, such as the radial artery. In addition, the lateral femoral cutaneous nerve can be preserved with the flap to make the flap sensate. The ALT flap may also be used as a pedicled flap for reconstructing the groin and perineum. The resulting donor-site scar from harvesting the LCFAP-*vl* flap is better accepted in oriental societies than in Western ones because of cultural and apparel differences.

The thoracodorsal artery perforator flap (T-DAP) described by Angrigiani in 1995[28] is a latissimus dorsi myocutaneous flap without the muscle component. The main perforators arise from the descending branch of the thoracodorsal vessel in the proximal free edge of the latissimus dorsi muscle. The perforators are few and far between, and the angiosomes are large in the posterior thorax. The angiosomes lie longitudinally; thus, a large flap can reliably be harvested on a small perforator. As a result of the paucity of perforators, preoperative duplex scanning is recommended.[29] The opportunity to preserve the largest muscle (latissimus dorsi) is hard to resist, and the T-DAP flap is growing in popularity. At present, the flap is used as a pedicled flap for reconstructing lateral breast defects after breast conservation surgery[30,31] and as a free flap for large defects requiring resurfacing.

A large number of other perforator flaps have been described. In some cases, dissecting a perforator flap might be easy, but when sacrificing a muscle does not leave any functional deficit, for example, as in a gracilis perforator flap, dissection may be unnecessary. At this moment, the size of the perforator vessels determines the number and size of skin flaps harvested. Flap harvest on very small vessels is technically very demanding, requiring much skill and specialist equipment to grasp the fine 12/0 sutures required to suture the 0.3 mm to 0.5 mm diameter perforator vessels.

Immediate thinning of perforator flaps allows the flap to be tailored to the defect at the time of initial surgery and may prevent the need for a secondary procedure. Such intraoperative debulking or "micro-lipectomy" requires knowing the exact location and branching of each perforator and due care if flap vascularity is not to be compromised.[20,32]

With the increasing safety and expertise of perforator-based surgery, an advanced form of flap harvest has developed that places even more priority on the donor site. In essence, free-style free flap surgery allows the surgeon to select the tissue characteristics most suited to the defect or a site preferred by the patient.[33] The donor area is mapped with the hand-held Doppler flow meter, and the perforator vessel is marked. The flap design is centred on the selected perforator. The tissue flap is raised supra- or sub-fascially as required, and the perforator vessel is dissected in a retrograde fashion until enough length or adequate vessel size is achieved. There are no anatomical limitations to dissection because either the intramuscular or septal course can be followed. Alternatively, without Doppler flowmetry, the surgeon may harvest a free-style free flap from a body site with which he or she is surgically familiar. Thus, a perforator flap may be harvested from the thigh, based on experience and knowledge of both the likely angiosome distribution and the usual location of suitable perforators.[33]

It may indeed be as Hallock predicts[34] that in the future, perforator-to-perforator free flaps and freestyle free flaps may make knowing the vascular origin or source vessel irrelevant because only the suprafascial location of the major perforators (>0.5 mm) mapped by Taylor and Palmer will be of any significance. Thus, the aphorism of Ecclesiastes that, "there is no new thing under the sun" will be confirmed. Once again, any skin paddle will be a potential donor site, and the underlying source vessel need not be known.

References

1. Blondeel PN, Van Landuyt KH, Monstrey SJ, et al. The "Gent" consensus on perforator flap terminology: preliminary definitions. *Plast Reconstr Surg.* 2003;112:1378–1383; quiz 1383, 1516; discussion 1384–1387.
2. Manchot C. *Die Hautarterien de Menschlichen Korpers.* Leipzig: F.C.W. Vogel, 1889.
3. Salmon M. *Arteres de la Peau.* Paris: Masson, 1936.
4. Esser JFS. General rules used in simple plastic work on Austrian war-wounded soldiers. *Surg Gynec Obstet.* 1917;34:737.
5. Milton SH. Pedicled skin-flaps: the fallacy of the length: width ratio. *Br J Surg.* 1970;57:502–508.
6. Bakamjian VY. A two stage method for pharyngo-oesophageal reconstruction with a primary pectoral skin flap. *Plast Reconstr Surg.* 1965;36:173–184.
7. McGregor IA, Morgan G. Axial and random pattern flaps. *Brit J Plast Surg.* 1973;26:202–213.
8. Taylor GI, Palmer JH. The vascular territories (angiosomes) of the body: experimental study and clinical applications. *Br J Plast Surg.* 1987;40:113–141.
9. Koshima I, Soeda S. Inferior epigastric artery skin flap without rectus abdominis muscle. *Brit J Plast Surg.* 1989;42:645–648.
10. Taylor GI. The angiosomes of the body and their supply to perforator flaps. In: Wei F-C, editor. *Clinics in Plastic Surgery, Vol. 30.* Philadelphia: W.B. Saunders, 2003.
11. Nakajima H, Fujino T, Adachi S. A new concept of vascular supply to the skin and classification of skin flaps according to their vascularization. *Ann Plast Surg.* 1986;16:1–19.
12. Blondeel PN, Van Landuyt K, Hamdi M, Monstrey SJ. Perforator flap terminology: update 2002. *Clin Plast Surg.* 2003;30:343–346, v.
13. Wei FC, Celik N. Perforator flap entity. *Clin Plast Surg.* 2003;30:325–329.
14. Blondeel PN, Beyens G, Verhaeghe R, et al. Doppler flowmetry in the planning of perforator flaps. *Br J Plast Surg.* 1998;51:202–209.
15. Blondeel PN. The sensate free superior gluteal artery perforator (S-GAP) flap: a valuable alternative in autologous breast reconstruction. *Br J Plast Surg.* 1999;52:185 193.
16. Kaplan JL, Allen RJ. Cost-based comparison between perforator flaps and TRAM flaps for breast reconstruction. *Plast Reconstr Surg.* 2000;105:943–48.
17. Kroll SS, Sharma S, Koutz C, et al. Postoperative morphine requirements of free TRAM and DIEP flaps. *Plast Reconstr Surg.* 2001;107:338–341.
18. Allen RJ, Treece P. Deep inferior epigastric perforator flap for breast reconstruction. *Ann Plast Surg.* 1994; 32:32–38.
19. Blondeel PN, Boeckx WD. Refinements in free flap breast reconstruction: the free bilateral deep inferior epigastric perforator flap anastomosed to the internal mammary artery. *Br J Plast Surg.* 1994;47:495–501.
20. Koshima I, Moriguchi T, Soeda S, Tanaka H, Umeda N. Free thin paraumbilical perforator-based flaps. *Ann Plast Surg.* 1992;29:12–17.
21. Koshima I, Inagawa K, Urushibara K, Moriguchi T. One-stage facial contour augmentation with intraoral transfer of a paraumbilical perforator adiposal flap. *Plast Reconstr Surg.* 2001;108:988–994.
22. Koshima I, Inagawa K, Yamamoto M, Moriguchi T. New microsurgical breast econstruction using free paraumbilical perforator adiposal flaps. *Plast Reconstr Surg.* 2000;106:61–65.
23. Blondeel N, Boeckx WD, Vanderstraeten GG, et al. The fate of the oblique abdominal muscles after free TRAM flap surgery. *Br J Plast Surg.* 1997;50: 315–321.
24. Futter CM, Webster MH, Hagen S, Mitchell SL. A retrospective comparison of abdominal muscle strength following breast reconstruction with a free TRAM or DIEP flap. *Br J Plast Surg.* 2000;53:578–583.
25. Futter CM, Weiler-Mithoff E, Hagen S, et al. Do preoperative abdominal exercises prevent post-operative donor site complications for women undergoing DIEP flap breast reconstruction? A two-centre, prospective randomised controlled trial. *Br J Plast Surg.* 2003;56: 674–683.
26. Koshima I, Moriguchi T, Soeda S, Kawata S, Ohta S, Ikeda A. The gluteal perforator-based flap for repair of sacral pressure sores. *Plast Reconstr Surg.* 1993;91: 678–683.
27. Song YG, Chen GZ, Song YL. The free thigh flap: a new free flap concept based on the septocutaneous artery. *Br J Plast Surg.* 1984;37:149–159.
28. Angrigiani C, Grilli D, Siebert J. Latissimus dorsi musculocutaneous flap without muscle. *Plast Reconstr Surg.* 1995;96:1608–1614.
29. Tonnard PL, Monstrey SJ, Van Landuyt KH, Blondeel PN, Matton GE. A simple mathematical formula for custom-made croissant tissue expanders. *Ann Plast Surg.* 1998;41:246–251.
30. Hamdi M, Van Landuyt K, Monstrey S, Blondeel P. Pedicled perforator flaps in breast reconstruction: a new concept. *Br J Plast Surg.* 2004;57:531–39.
31. Van Landuyt K, Hamdi M, Blondeel P, Monstrey S. Autologous breast augmentation by pedicled perforator flaps. *Ann Plast Surg.* 2004;53:322–327.
32. Koshima I, Saisho H, Kawada S, Hamanaka T, Umeda N, Moriguchi T. Flow through thin latissimus dorsi perforator flap for repair of soft-tissue defects in the legs. *Plast Reconstr Surg.* 1999;103:1483–1490.
33. Mardini S, Tsai FC, Wei FC. The thigh as a model for free style free flaps. *Clin Plast Surg.* 2003;30:473–480.
34. Hallock GG. Direct and indirect perforator flaps: the history and the controversy. *Plast Reconstr Surg.* 2003;111:855–865; quiz 866.

8

Remote Ischemic Preconditioning of Flaps: Current Concepts

Markus V. Küntscher, Bernd Hartmann and Günter Germann

Introduction

Ischemic preconditioning (IP) of a flap is defined as a brief period of ischemia ("preclamping") followed by tissue reperfusion that increases the tolerance of the flap for a subsequent longer ischemic period. Several studies have showed the effectiveness of classic local IP by preclamping the flap pedicle.

There are two temporally and mechanically different types of IP: acute preconditioning, which is induced by preclamping the flap pedicle briefly before flap ischemia, and late preconditioning, which is induced by a preclamping procedure 24 to 48 hours before flap ischemia. However, neither type of IP is commonly used clinically, most likely because they are invasive, substantially increase surgical time, or even require a second surgery.

We have shown in different experimental models that acute IP, enhancement of flap survival, and improved microvascular reperfusion can be achieved not only by preclamping the flap pedicle, but also by inducing an ischemia-reperfusion event in a body area distant from the flap before elevation. This new, acute "remote ischemia preconditioning" procedure can be applied noninvasively by applying a tourniquet shortly before flap ischemia. The effectiveness of acute remote IP has been confirmed by other authors in large animal models.

The use of a tourniquet to induce limb ischemia before flap ischemia could provide a new, alternative, noninvasive remote IP protocol, although late remote IP might be effective only in muscle flaps. However, the possible future clinical application for late IP is elective flap surgery, whereas acute remote IP could even be used to create emergency flaps.

Historical Preface

Although the word *plastic* is derived from the Greek word *plastikos*, meaning "to mold" or "to give form," the true origins of the modern specialty of plastic and reconstructive surgery predate even this archaic linguistic root. Some historians trace the foundations of the specialty as far back as the early papyri of Egypt and the Sanskrit texts of ancient India. Within these early Hindu texts, possibly written more than 2600 years ago, lie descriptions of nose, ear, and lip reconstructions using techniques ranging from pedicle flaps to free autogenous skin grafts.[1-3]

Hellenistic, Roman, and Byzantine physicians developed further basic reconstructive principles and techniques, such as tensionless suture lines, the débridement of exposed bone, and the use of flaps to avoid the distortion of facial features associated with primary closure, bipedicle advancement flaps for facial defects, undermining tissues before wound closure, the risk of necrosis if the skin alone was undermined, and the first superiorly based nasolabial flap.[1,4]

Despite continued use of established methods, the fall of Rome in the fifth century and the subsequent spread of barbarian tribes and Christianity throughout the Middle Ages brought an unfortunate halt in the advancement of reconstructive surgery. The atmosphere of the time was apparent in the 13th century, when Pope Innocent III specifically prohibited surgical procedures. The advent of the Renaissance in the 14th century brought a rebirth of science and medicine and an end to the stagnation that had befallen the world of surgery. Gasparo Tagliacozzi introduced the principles and use of distant pedicle flaps and carefully detailed the delayed arm flap for nose reconstruction in the "Italian Method" during the second half of the 16th century.[1,5,6]

The modern era of reconstructive plastic surgery was strongly influenced by a simple letter, published in 1791 in a London gentleman's magazine, by a British surgeon named Lucas, on nasal reconstruction using an Indian forehead flap.[7] Vilray Papin Blair, Sir Harold Delf Gillies, and other physicians during World Wars I and II initiated modern reconstructive surgery by introducing cross-leg flaps, tube flaps, and delayed transfer of long pedicle flaps.[8,9]

The development of micro instruments, fine suture material, and the binocular operating microscope by the Carl-Zeiss Company in the mid-1950s revolutionized the field of plastic and reconstructive surgery and lead to the birth of microsurgery. From this time on, plastic surgeons were no longer limited to local pedicled flaps and soon developed microvascular tissue transplantation. Soon, several new microvascular flaps were introduced, including the first autologous transfer of omentum by Donald McLean in 1969, the first free temporal skin flap by Harii and Ohmori in 1972,[10] the free latissimus dorsi flap by Olivari in 1976,[11] and the free transverse rectus abdominis flap by Holström in 1979,[12] among many others.

This historical overview documents an increase in complexity and variety of reconstructive procedures over time. However, the introduction of the axial pattern pedicle and free flaps or even the latest innovation of perforator based flaps[13-17] are associated with higher risks for flap necrosis as a result of ischemia or reperfusion injury. This risk emphasizes the necessity to explore acute and late flap preconditioning.

Ischemia Reperfusion Injury

Tissue ischemia and reperfusion involve complex mechanisms that have not yet been completely identified or understood. However, reperfusing tissues after acute ischemia initiates changes in local vascular tone, coagulation, and biochemical, molecular, and cellular alterations that are collectively called "ischemia-reperfusion injury."[18,19] The activation of neutrophil granulocytes by oxygen-free radicals and consecutive

endothelial injury are the central processes in ischemia-reperfusion injury.[20,21] Neutrophil activation and up-regulation of corresponding receptors in the postcapillary venules leads to adhesions between white cells and endothelium, which can be visualized by in-vivo microscopy as leukocyte "sticking" and "rolling." Segmental vessel occlusion occurs as a result of this leukocyte-endothelium interaction, leading to leukocyte migration into tissue, increased production of oxygen-free radicals, and tissue-damaging enzymes. The lack of venous reflow occurs in tissues after prolonged ischemia and is caused by irreversible capillary damage and total or subtotal vascular occlusion.[22,23] Finally, cell death occurs as a result of the influx of potassium, mediators, and oxygen-free radicals, as well as through decreased intracellular ATP concentrations and hypoxia.[24]

Reperfusion of ischemic tissues is essential for survival, although it augments tissue damage induced by ischemia. Therefore, it is also termed "reflow paradox."[18,25]

The Delay Procedure

In rats, transverse rectus abdominis musculocutaneous (TRAM) flaps survived longer after surgical delay.[26] In related research, Restifo et al. reported an increase in mean vessel diameter and superior epigastric artery flow in 15 patients 1 week after a preliminary TRAM flap delay.[27] These findings are consistent with previous anatomic studies by Taylor and colleagues, who reported that the arterial choke vessel system dilated in the rectus muscle and that venous valve incompetence allowed venous drainage toward the superior epigastric system.[28] These data were confirmed in other clinical studies.[30,31]

Surgical delay (skin incision down to fascia) should be distinguished from pure vascular delay (ligation of one of the dominant vessels of a type-3 muscle according to Mathes and Nahai's classification.[31,32] TRAM flap delay has been promoted 7 days, 2 weeks, and up to 1 month before flap transfer.

The delay phenomenon has widely been used clinically to improve flap survival in the distal portion of axial pattern flaps, but its main disadvantages are the need for a second surgical procedure and anesthesia and thus additional costs for both health system and patients.

Classic Local Ischemic Preconditioning ("Preclamping")

Murry et al. were the first to describe IP or "preclamping" for the heart in 1986.[33] Similar results have been reported for other organ systems, such as the liver[34] and the kidney.[35] Various studies report the success of IP in flaps.[36–40] Mounsey et al., were the first to report this phenomenon in a porcine latissimus dorsi flap model in 1992.[37] Caroll et al. observed in a rat latissimus dorsi model that IP, both immediately preoperatively and 24 hours before flap ischemia, significantly reduced muscle flap necrosis.[36] Another study reported the influence of ischemic preconditioning on the resistance of skin and myocutaneous flaps after long ischemic periods in a rat model.[40] Critical ischemia time, the time at which 50% of the flap becomes necrotic, is prolonged significantly by preconditioning. Vasospasm and lack of capillary reflow was attenuated by acute ischemic preconditioning in an in vivo microscopic study of rat cremaster muscle flaps.[38,39]

Total necrosis in flaps is rare and is usually found only after vascular thrombosis of the pedicle or prolonged ischemic periods. Moreover, it is most probably not preventable by ischemic preconditioning. On the other hand, partial flap necrosis or fat tissue necrosis occurs in up to 30% of certain flaps, such as the pedicle TRAM.[27,41] These complications could be potentially decreased by IP. Most recent studies report significant reduction in the extent of flap necrosis in standard models. However, classic local IP has rarely been used clinically,[27] most likely because it significantly increases operative time and is invasive.

Remote Ischemic Preconditioning

In 1993, Przyklenk et al. first observed that regional IP of the heart not only protects those myocytes subjected to brief coronary occlusion from ischemia-reperfusion injury but also limits infarct size in remote "virgin" myocardium in a canine model.[42] Verdouw et al. were the first to report a real remote IP of the heart by mesenteric artery occlusion in a rat model.[43] The protective influence of limb ischemia on myocardial infarction has also been reported by Birnbaum et al. and Oxman et al.[44,45]

We showed in a rat adipocutaneous flap model that acute IP and flap survival can be enhanced not only by preclamping the flap pedicle but also by inducing an ischemia—reperfusion event in a body area distant from the flap before elevation.[46] An invasive procedure, clamping the femoral artery is as effective at preconditioning the flap as a noninvasive tourniquet applied to the rat hind limb followed by 30 minutes limb reperfusion (Figures 8-1 and 8-2). A second study focusing on remote IP of skeletal muscle showed that both classic and remote acute IP improved microcirculation of muscle flaps after ischemia.[47] Both preconditioning protocols improved red blood cell velocity in the arterioles and capillaries, improved capillary flow (Figure 8-3a), and decreased neutrophil accumulation in the postcapillary venules (Figure 8-3b).

Capillary no-reflow and leukocyte-endothelial adhesions are the central microcirculatory patterns that determine the severity of ischemia-reperfusion injury in the cremaster model. The number of temporarily adhering leukocytes (rollers) did not differ significantly in any of the experimental groups in our series (Figure 8-4). These findings might be to the result of a shorter ischemic period than used by other authors.[38,39] However, in our opinion, an ischemic period of 4 hours is rare in a clinical setting, so we, as have others,[48] used 2 hours of ischemia in our experiments. In contrast to other authors,[38,39,48] we used a microvascular clamp directly on the flap pedicle to prevent additional limb ischemia, which always occurs when clamping a segment of

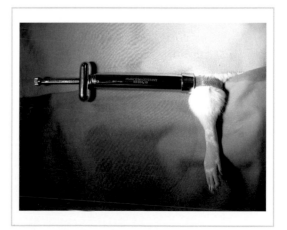

Figure 8-1. A noninvasive tourniquet (Martin, Tuttlingen, Germany) applied to the hind limb of a rat to induce ischemia.

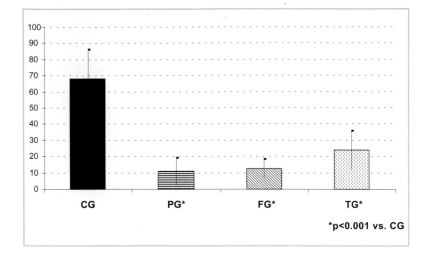

Figure 8-2. Clamping the femoral artery is as effective at preconditioning the flap as a noninvasive tourniquet applied to the rat hind limb followed by 30 minutes limb reperfusion.[27] Average flap necrosis was 68.2% (±18.1%) in the control group (CG), 11 ± 8.38% in the preclamping group (PG), 12.5 ± 5.83% in the femoral ischemic group (FG), and 24 ± 11.75% in the tourniquet group (TG). All preconditioned animals had a significantly smaller area of flap necrosis than did the control animals (*p < 0.001 vs. CG). The differences between PG, FG and TG groups were not significant.

the femoral artery and vein. Short-term limb ischemia has a preconditioning effect on flaps.[46,47] Thus, longer-term limb ischemia might also influence flap ischemia—reperfusion injury.

Recently, Addison et al.[49] confirmed our data on the effectiveness of noninvasive acute remote IP for global protection of skeletal muscle against ischemic necrosis in a large animal model. Three 10-minute cycles of occlusion and reperfusion in a pig hind limb using a tourniquet significantly reduced infarctions of the latissimus dorsi, gracilis, and rectus abdominis muscles by 55%, 60%, and 55%, respectively, compared to a control group. Whether remote ischemic preconditioning could be induced by a late mechanism was also determined.[50] A rat hind limb was subjected to 10 minutes of ischemia and 30 minutes of reperfusion with a tourniquet 24 hours before flap ischemia. This protocol increased red blood cell velocity in the capillaries and first-order arterioles and venules and increased capillary flow, as well as decreased leukocyte sticking in a cremaster model and thus, attenuated early ischemia-reperfusion injury in muscle flaps. On the other hand, it did not improve flap survival in adipocutaneous flaps. These findings indicate

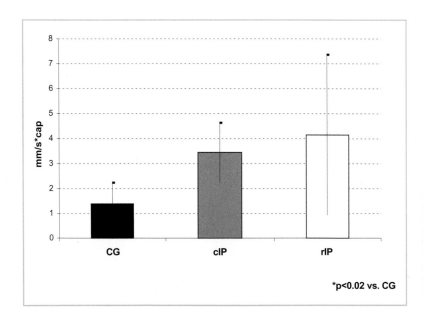

Figure 8-3. Both classic and remote acute ischemic preconditioning improve microcirculation of muscle flaps after ischemia in a rat model.[47] Capillary flow results; capillary flow was significantly higher in the groups with classic ischemic preconditioning (cIP) and remote ischemic preconditioning (rIP) than in the control group (p < 0.02). The difference within the groups cIP and rIP was not significant.

16.

17.

18.

19.

20.

21.

22.

23.

24.

25.

26.

27.

28.

29.

30.

31.

32.

33.

34.

35

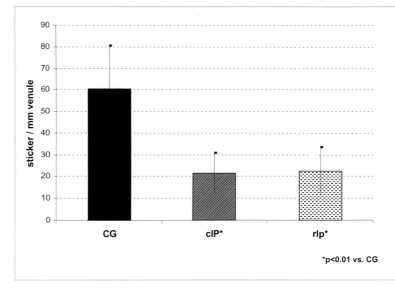

Figure 8-4. Leukocyte count. A significantly lower number of permanent adhering leucocytes (stickers) was observed in both the preconditioned groups cIP and rIP, compared to the control group (p < 0.01).

that acute and late remote IP are induced by different mechanisms.

A few studies have focused on the possible mechanisms of remote IP. Takaoka et al. investigated the involvement of adenosine receptors in the mechanism of remote IP of the heart by renal ischemia. The improvement of myocardial energy metabolism induced by classic and remote IP was abolished in rabbits by blocking adenosine receptors.[51] Dickson et al. postulated that remote IP is initiated by a humoral mechanism because the venous effluent from a preconditioned heart of a donor rabbit, transfused to an recipient animal, lead to the same effect as "preclamping" in a control group.[52] In contrast, Schoemaker and van Heijningen observed that antagonizing the bradykinin 2 receptor abolished the protective effect of remote cardiac IP, whereas a simulation of bradykinin release by local intra-arterial infusion could mimic remote IP in a rat model. These results support the hypothesis that remote IP acts through sensory nerve stimulation in ischemic organs.[53]

Our data show that ischemic preconditioning and enhancement of flap survival can be achieved not only by preclamping the flap pedicle but also by inducing an ischemia—reperfusion event in a body area distant from the flap before elevation. These findings indicate that remote IP in flaps must be a systemic phenomenon and not merely a local reaction in the flap itself.

The Role of Nitric Oxide in Preconditioning

The exact mechanism of classic as well as remote IP is not yet determined. Two temporally and mechanistically distinct types of protection are induced by preconditioning stimuli: acute and delayed.[54,55] Various factors, such as nitric oxide (NO),[55,56] heat shock proteins,[57–59] adenosine,[60,61] ATP-sensitive K+ channels,[62] cyclooxygenase-2,[63] or bradykinin through sensory nerve stimulation,[53] seem to be involved in ischemic preconditioning. However, the protective effects of acute preconditioning are independent of protein synthesis, whereas delayed preconditioning requires de novo protein synthesis.[55]

Nitric oxide may be central to the mechanism of ischemic preconditioning. Peralta et al. found in a rat model of hepatic ischemia-reperfusion that adenosine or NO administration before ischemia simulated the effect of preconditioning, whereas inhibition of NO synthesis eliminated the protective effect of hepatic preconditioning.[64] We confirmed these data in two studies of adipocutaneous[65] and muscle[66] flaps. In contrast to our data, Peralta et al. observed a continuing protective effect of exogenous NO after endogenous NO synthesis was blocked by NG-Nitro-L-arginine-methyl ester hydrochloride (L-NAME). We found that exogenous NO, in a dose similar to that used by Peralta et al., did not enhance flap survival after L-NAME administration. A

receptors in rabbits: effects of "remote preconditioning" *J Am Coll Cardiol.* 1999;33(2):556–64.

52. Dickson EW, Lorbar M, Porcaro WA, et al. Rabbit heart can be "preconditioned" via transfer of coronary effluent. *Am J Physiol.* 1999;277(6 Pt 2):H2451–2457.

53. Schoemaker RG, van Heijningen CL. Bradykinin mediates cardiac preconditioning at a distance. *Am J Physiol Heart Circ Physiol.* 2000;278(5):H1571–1576.

54. Dawn B, Bolli R. Toward a better understanding of the metabolic effects of ischemic preconditioning in humans. *J Cardiothorac Vasc Anesth.* 2001;15(4): 409–411.

55. Nandagopal K, Dawson TM, Dawson VL. Critical role for nitric oxide signaling in cardiac and neuronal ischemic preconditioning and tolerance. *J Pharmacol Exp Ther.* 2001;297(2):474–478.

56. Peralta C, Hotter G, Closa D, Gelpí E, Bulbena O, Roselló-Catafau J. Protective effect of preconditioning on the injury associated to hepatic ischemia-reperfusion in the rat: role of nitric oxide and adenosine. *Hepatology.* 1997;25:934–937.

57. Kume M, Yamamoto Y, Saad S, et al. Ischemic preconditioning of the liver in rats: Implications of heat shock protein induction to increase tolerance of ischemia-reperfusion injury. *J Lab Clin Med.* 1996;128: 251–258.

58. Lille S, Su CY, Schoeller T, et al. Induction of heat-shock protein 72 in rat skeletal muscle does not increase tolerance to ischemia-reperfusion injury. *Muscle Nerve.* 1999;22:390–393.

59. Wang BH, Ye C, Stagg CA, et al. Improved free musculocutaneous flap survival with induction of heat shock protein. *Plast Reconstr Surg.* 1998;101(3):776–784.

60. Pang CY, Neligan P, Zhong A, He W, Xu H, Forrest CR. Effector mechanism of adenosine in acute ischemic preconditioning of skeletal muscle against infarction. *Am J Physiol.* 1997;273:R887–895.

61. Yokota R, Fujiwara H, Miyamae M, et al. Transient adenosine infusion before ischemia and reperfusion protects against metabolic damage in pig hearts. *Am J Physiol.* 1995;268:H1149–1157.

62. Pang CY, Neligan P, Xu H, et al. Role of ATP-sensitive K+ channels in ischemic preconditioning of skeletal muscle against infarction. *Am J Physiol.* 1997;273: H44–51.

63. Guo Y, Bao W, Wu WJ, Shinmura K, Tang XL, Bolli R. Evidence for an essential role of cyclooxygenase-2 as a mediator of the late phase of ischemic preconditioning in mice. *Basic Res Cardiol.* 2000;95(6):479–484.

64. Peralta C, Closa D, Hotter G, Gelpí E, Prats N, Roselló-Catafau J. Liver ischemic preconditioning is mediated by the inhibitory action of nitric oxide on endothelin. *Biochem Biophys Res Comm.* 1996;229: 271–274.

65. Küntscher MV, Juran S, Altmann J, Menke H, Gebhard MM, Germann G. The role of nitric oxide in the mechanism of preclamping and remote ischemic preconditioning of flaps in a rat model. *J Reconstr Microsurg.* 2003;19(1):55–60.

66. Küntscher MV, Kastell T, Altmann J, Menke H, Gebhard MM, Germann G. Acute remote ischemic preconditioning II: the role of nitric oxide. *Microsurgery.* 2002;22(6):227–231.

67. Chen JX, Berry LC, Tanner M, Chang M, Myers RP, Meyrick B. Nitric oxide donors regulate nitric oxide synthase in bovine pulmonary artery endothelium. *J Cell Physiol.* 2001;186(1):116–123.

68. Rakhit RD, Edwards RJ, Marber MS. Nitric oxide, nitrates and ischaemic preconditioning. *Cardiovasc Res.* 1999;43(3):621–627.

69. Cordeiro PG, Santamaria E, Hu QY. Use of a nitric oxide precursor to protect pig myocutaneous flaps from ischemia-reperfusion injury. *Plast Reconstr Surg.* 1998; 102:2040–2048; discussion, 2049–2051.

70. Küntscher MV, Juran S, Menke H, Gebhard MM, Erdmann D, Germann G. The role of pre-ischaemic application of the nitric oxide donor spermine/nitric oxide complex in enhancing flap survival in a rat model. *Br J Plast Surg.* 2002;55(5):430–433.

71. Ghaleh B, Tissier R, Berdeaux A. Nitric oxide and myocardial ischemic preconditioning. *J Soc Biol.* 2000;194(3–4):137–141.

72. Jones WK, Flaherty MP, Tang XL, Takano H, Qiu Y, Banerjee S, et al. Ischemic preconditioning increases iNOS transcript levels in conscious rabbits via a nitric oxide-dependent mechanism. *J Mol Cell Cardiol.* 1999;31(8):1469–1481.

73. Wang WZ, Anderson GL, Guo SZ, Tsai TM, Miller FN. Initiation of microvascular protection by nitric oxide in late preconditioning. *J Reconstr Microsurg.* 2000;16(8):621–628.

74. Oshima H. The influence of skin flap ischemia on serum nitric oxide concentrations. *Microsurgery.* 1996;17(4): 191–197.

9

Advances in Facial Aesthetic Surgery: New Approaches to Old Problems and Current Approaches to New Problems

James E. Zins and Andrea Moreira-Gonzalez

Introduction

As our lives become forever more hectic, men and women in the United States are becoming more time conscious and less accepting of surgical procedures requiring prolonged recovery. This circumstance has led to increasing attention being paid to lesser or minimally invasive procedures rather than traditional ones. The media, the Internet, and television shows have popularized many of these techniques. Although some of these techniques may be effective, many have not been held to strict scientific rigor.

The recent popularity of surgical procedures for the correction of massive weight loss has markedly increased the popularity and incidence of plastic surgery procedures for correcting skin excess. In fact, plastic surgery correction for patients who have undergone bariatric surgery is predicted to be one of the fastest-growing areas of plastic surgery in the ensuing years. Aesthetic facial correction in these patients requires special considerations and variations on current techniques.

Finally, although new treatments for HIV/AIDS have prolonged survival, they have also resulted in a new group of patients with facial deformities that are amenable to plastic surgery correction.

Here, we review the above topics and our preferred methods for treating them.

Browlift

Endoscopic surgery came relatively late to plastic surgery. The endoscopic browlift was introduced in 1995, long after endoscopic procedures were commonplace in general surgery, gynecologic surgery, and other surgical subspecialties. Vasconez was the first to popularize the endoscopic browlift when he realized that an "optical cavity" could be developed through a subperiosteal forehead dissection.[1,2] The procedure was soon popularized by others and since has become widely accepted.[3-10] Most surgeons favor the subperiosteal approach, but the subgaleal approach is preferred by others.[11-14]

The endoscopic approach differs conceptually from the traditional coronal or hairline browlift. The endoscopic approach depends not on mechanical elevation by skin or scalp excision but on weakening the antagonistic affect of the depressor muscles of the forehead (the corrugators, procerus, and orbicularis oculi). This weakening of the depressors allows the forehead elevator (frontalis) to function with less opposition, resulting in brow elevation. Critical to the success of the subperiosteal browlift are the following prerequisites:

1. Wide release of the arcus marginalis or periosteum of the supraorbital rim, the superior temporal line, and the temporal ligament
2. Alteration by resection of the depressor muscles of the forehead, allowing the frontalis to work relatively unopposed
3. Adequate (predominantly lateral) fixation of the forehead soft tissues

Conversely, pitfalls include inadequate release of the arcus marginalis, inadequate muscle excision, and inadequate fixation. Common postoperative problems, therefore, include the following:

1. Undercorrection of brow elevation, especially laterally. This lack of adequate lateral elevation results predominantly from inadequate lateral soft tissue release or inadequate fixation.

2. Overcorrection of the brow medially. Overcorrection medially results from improper surgical planning and is the direct result of corrugator resection.

3. Recurrence of corrugator hyperactivity resulting from inadequate corrugator resection.

In other words, it may be the surgeon who fails the patient, rather than the procedure that leads to less-than-ideal results.

Proper patient selection is also critical if pleasing results are to be obtained. Certain patients with brow ptosis are clearly not good candidates for the endoscopic browlift. Such patients have high hairlines or marked or severe eyebrow ptosis. The patient with the high hairline is better addressed by a traditional hairline browlift incision, rather than by a pure endoscopic approach. If the hairline incision is used, the hairline can be lowered, in addition to the brow being elevated, thereby shortening the forehead and giving the patient a more youthful appearance. Alternatively, the hairline and an endoscopic

approach can be combined, as described by Ramirez.[3,4] The patient with a heavy brow and severe brow ptosis is probably best approached by excisional surgery to maximize forehead elevation.

Means of fixation have also evolved over the past 10 years. Early endoscopic approaches used bolster dressings, sutures or, more commonly, percutaneous screw fixation.[6,11] The percutaneous screw was placed through the lateral endobrow incision and into the outer table of the skull. A staple was then used behind the screw to maintain forehead elevation, once the scalp and forehead had been pulled posteriorly. Although effective, this approach resulted in traction on the scalp that occasionally caused hair loss. Further, patients were quite averse to the exposed screws in their scalp and were displeased at the idea of having screws in their skulls.

Percutaneous screws have been replaced by other techniques, including resorbable plates, screws and suture, the Endotine device, or the cortical-tunnel technique.[15–18] We use the

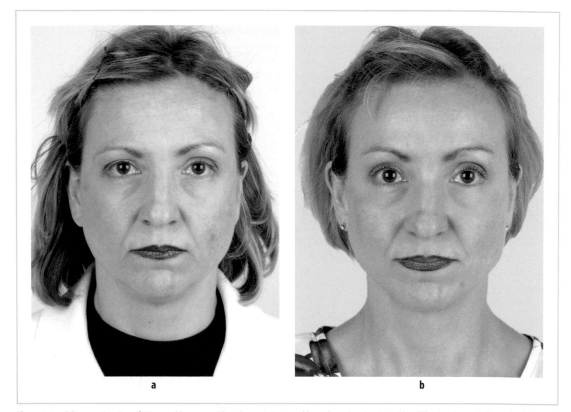

Figure 9-1. a) Preoperative view of 43-year-old woman with eyebrow ptosis treated by endoscopic subperiosteal browlift using the cortical tunnel technique for fixation, a cheeklift, and submental liposuction. **b)** The patient 1 year later.

cortical-tunnel technique, from craniofacial surgery. Oblique holes are drilled in an anterior and posterior direction through the lateral scalp incision used during the endoscopic approach. A suture is passed through this cortical tunnel, the forehead flap is grasped from its deep surface, and the suture is tied. The cortical tunnel can be drilled very superficially and, thus, penetration of the inner table avoided. The skull in this area may be only 7 mm or 8 mm thick.[19] The cortical technique is fast, easily accomplished, and requires no expensive devices. Fixation is applied laterally only and, again, it is difficult to overcorrect laterally and easy to overcorrect medially. Intraoperative time required for drilling of the tunnel is 3 minutes. We have had no complications with the cortical tunnel in more than 100 cases (Figure 9-1).

Midface Correction

Interest in correcting defects of the midface began in the early 1990s and has continued since. Standard facelift approaches for correcting the mid face in the sub-SMAS plane, the subperiosteal plane, and the subcutaneous plane, have all been recommended. Virtually all modern sub-SMAS facelift procedures that provide adequate midface correction involve releasing the major zygomatic cutaneous ligament and the upper masseteric cutaneous ligaments, with or without malar fat pad repositioning.[20-29] These procedures differ in the amount of skin undermining, the method of fixating mobilized midface structures, and the manipulation of the malar fat pad.

An extension of the endoscopic browlift approach for midface correction has been popularized by a number of authors.[30-33] These authors use either the subperiosteal [30-33] or the subgaleal approach.[8]

Although classically described as ineffective in the long-term, "spanning sutures" have gained in popularity. Little's facelift technique makes use of such sutures and is conceptually appealing.[34-35] Little combines an endoscopic approach from the temporal area with intraoral exposure of the maxilla. After temporal dissection, he makes an intraoral incision and exposes the maxilla, the piriform aperture, and the zygomatic eminence. Then, through the intraoral route, he places a suture on the line intersecting

the lateral canthus vertically, with a line drawn horizontally from the alar base. At the intersection of these two lines, he grasps the soft tissue from the intraoral approach, on the undersurface of the cheek soft tissue. This spanning suture is then passed through the mouth to the temporal incision and sewn to the temporalis fascia proper. A standard facelift incision is then made after the above incisions are closed. An extended subcutaneous facelift is then followed by horizontal placation of the soft tissues in the lower face.[34-35]

Vasconez has taken a different approach.[36-37] He approaches the malar fat pad and elevates the midface through an anterior hairline subcutaneous approach. Through this approach, the malar fat pad is exposed, with dissection extending medially toward the nasolabial fold. The malar fat pad is then grasped through the subcutaneous dissection, along the vertical line corresponding to the level of the lateral canthus. Several spanning sutures are then placed through the malar fat pad, directed superiorly and posteriorly, and attached to the intermediate temporal fascia. Although this approach is effective, the drawback is that the anterior hairline incision may become visible. More recently, Vasconez recommended this procedure predominantly for elderly patients, who would be more accepting of this anterior incision.

Hester's approach to the midface has been a subperiosteal approach through a lower eyelid incision.[38] For the past 10 years, the Hester group has gained vast experience with the subperiosteal lower eyelid approach and has varied their technique a number of times. Their current technique is that of a lower eyelid, subperiosteal, endoscopically assisted approach to the midface. Careful attention to lateral canthus support and conservative resection of the lower eyelid skin is critical to their results.[39] The learning curve to this procedure is well recognized, and experience is necessary to avoid lower eyelid complications.

Our approach to the midface is similar to Little's. In the younger patient, we combine the endoscopic temporal approach with the intraoral approach and avoid the facelift component of the operation (Figure 9-2). This combination gives consistent, adequate midface elevation without lower eyelid complications. The operation is not complication-free, however. Transient buccal-branch weakness occurs in approximately 15% of our patients. To ensure adequate release

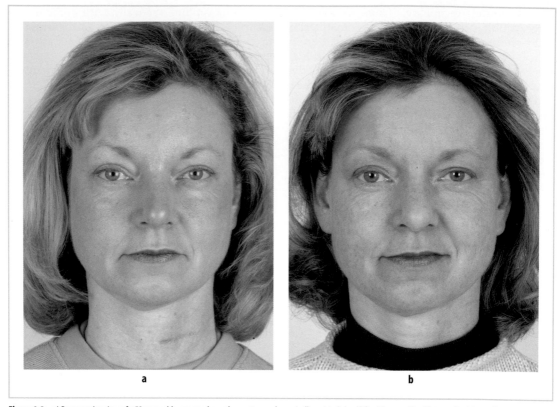

Figure 9-2. a) Preoperative view of a 52-year-old woman who underwent an endoscopically assisted cheeklift, with a combined intraoral incision and spanning sutures from the intraoral soft tissues to the temporalis fascia proper. **b**) The patient 1 year later.

through the intraoral approach, we stretch the soft tissues of the cheek with an index finger placed through the intraoral incision. This stretching is the probable cause of the buccal nerve neuropraxia. In addition, soft tissue infection, presumably related to the combined intraoral and temporal approaches, occurs in about 10% of our patients.

To minimize recovery time, minimally invasive suture techniques have been developed, including the minimal access cranial suspension (MACS-lift), barbed sutures, and the endoscopically assisted cheek lift using the Endotine midface device (Coapt Co.).[16,40] The surgical outcomes of these techniques have not been published; however, at least one study documents substantial complications with the barbed sutures.[41]

In summary, spanning techniques work best in younger patients. Complications can include asymmetry, transient buccal nerve weakness, and infection.

Perioral Rejuvenation

The perioral area has also received increasing attention in recent years. This area is often inadequately addressed by cervicofacial rhytidectomy alone. Aging of the perioral area is exacerbated by a number of factors related to both bone and soft tissue. Perhaps most important is the loss of the alveolar ridge and tooth support.[42] Tooth loss leads to alveolar ridge resorption, mandibular overclosure reduced vertical facial height, and maxillary retrusion. With a lack of support, the upper lip lengthens like a curtain, and the vermilion inverts. Correcting these problems requires a maxillofacial prosthodontic approach, including denture fabrication alone or combined with bone grafting and osseointegrated implant techniques.

With the development of skin laxity, vertical rhytids begin to appear, at first only with animation. As aging continues, the vertical lines become present at rest. These vertical rhytids reflect the perpendicular ligamentous attachments from the orbicularis oris and the muscle to dermis. They are clearly more common in women and rarely seen in men. Further vertical rhytids are more common in Fitzpatrick I and II female skin types. We presume, without proof, that this increased frequency is the result of a decrease in the subcutaneous tissue of the upper lip in the Fitzpatrick I and II female skin types.

The downturn of the corners of the mouth is a common complaint of women with facial aging. This downturn is difficult to correct with a face-lift alone. Clearly, the most effective pull is accomplished where skin laxity is the greatest; that is, a direct browlift is more effective than a coronal browlift for the correcting brow ptosis. Therefore, only 1 cm of skin need be excised to elevate the brow 1 cm with a direct browlift, whereas 2 cm to 2.5 cm of scalp needs to be excised for every centimeter of eyebrow elevation in a coronal browlift. Similarly, adjusting the downturned corners of the mouth at the level of the commissure is a mechanically more effective than correcting the downturn through a facelift incision.

Excisional and nonexcisional techniques have been used to correct the effects of aging on the perioral area. These techniques are employed with or without a variety of resurfacing methods. External incisional techniques include shortening the lip with a gull-wing excision at the alar base to correct the long upper lip; enhancing the vermilion by excising the upper lip at the vermilion-cutaneous junction and advancing the vermilion (Figure 9-3); and lifting the corner of the lip to correct the downturned corners of the mouth (Figure 9-4).[43–50]

The obvious drawback of these techniques is the external scar that may be aesthetically unacceptable. In our experience, CO_2 laser resurfacing over the scar at the time of excisional surgery greatly reduces the visibility of the scar.

With regard to shortening the upper lip, certain precepts should be followed. The ideal patient for lip shortening has an aging face in which the length of the upper lip is greater than the vertical distance from the commissure to the soft tissue menton, with a decrease in upper incisor show. If upper incisor show is less than 3 mm, vertical shortening with a gull-wing incision will reduce the edentulous look and enhance the appearance of the lower face. However, if upper incisor show is already normal, further upper lip skin excision will create the appearance of vertical maxillary excess and, therefore, should be avoided. In addition, those patients who already have an arched appearance of the upper lip are not candidates for shortening of the upper lip because shortening will enhance the arched appearance and create an unnatural result.

A corner-of-the-lip lift, as popularized by Austin and Westin, will correct the downturned corners of the mouth.[44] This technique is

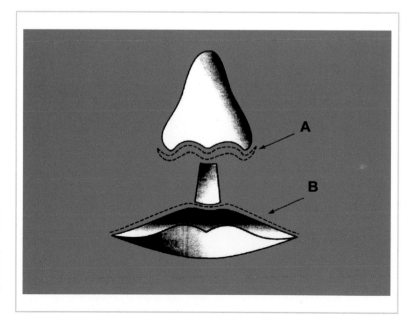

Figure 9-3. The gull-wing excision at the base of the nose to shorten the upper lip and lip-lift procedure by direct excision of skin above the vermilion-cutaneous junction. (Reprinted from Plastic Surgery 2/e, Mathes SJ, chapter: Face Lift (Lower Face): Current Techniques by Fardo D, Zins JE, Nahai F, ©2005 Elsevier Inc. With permission from Elsevier.)

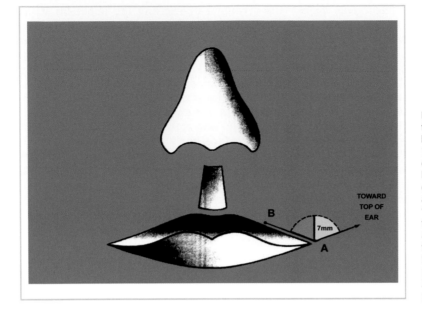

Figure 9-4. **a)** Corner of the lip lift performed by marking the commissure. **b)** Drawing a line from the commissure 11 mm long medially along the vermilion-cutaneous junction and drawing a second line from "A" laterally toward the top of the ear. These lines create a triangle with the apex of the triangle at "A" and the base at "B-C." The vertical distance from "A" is 5 mm for minimal lip elevation, 7 mm for moderate elevation (most common), and 9 mm for high elevation. (Reprinted from Plastic Surgery 2/e, Mathes SJ, chapter: Face Lift (Lower Face): Current Techniques by Fardo D, Zins JE, Nahai F, ©2005 Elsevier Inc. With permission from Elsevier.)

performed by first identifying and marking the commissure. A line is then drawn medially along the vermilion for approximately 11 mm long, and a second line is drawn from the commissure laterally towards the top of the ear. The triangle thus created by connecting these two lines should have a base of 5 mm (if minimal elevation is required), 7 mm (for moderate elevation), or 9 mm (for marked elevation).[43,44] The triangle is then closed as a straight line, correcting the downturned corners of the mouth (Figure 9-5).

Nonexcisional correction of perioral aging can be performed by autologous or nonautologous fillers. Fat grafting, as popularized by Coleman, has become by far the most common autologous procedure for soft tissue augmentation. Coleman has had excellent results with fat injection for lip augmentation, correction of the marionette lines, chin augmentation, and prejowl augmentation. Although Coleman obtains consistently excellent results, others find these results difficult to reproduce. Coleman's success appears to be the result of meticulous technique. Most importantly, he injects small amounts of fat through many tunnels at various levels of the skin and soft tissue envelope.[51,52]

In non-autologous volume augmentation, hyaluronic acid (Restylane, Medicis Pharmaceu-

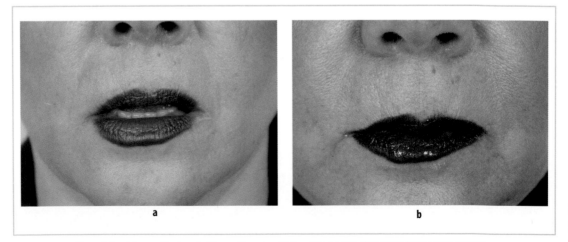

Figure 9-5. **a)** Preoperative view of a 59-year-old woman with downturned corners of the mouth. **b)** The patient 1 year later.

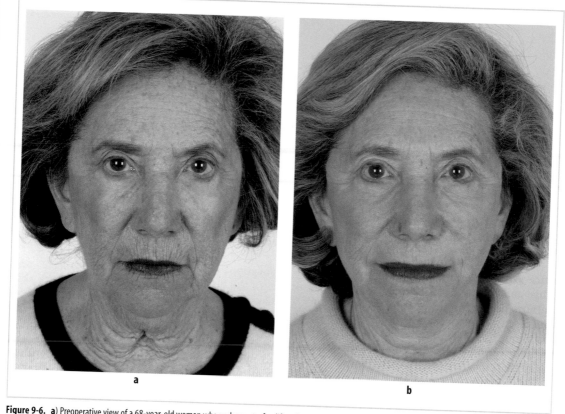

Figure 9-6. **a**) Preoperative view of a 68-year-old woman who underwent a facelift and perioral phenol-croton oil peel using 50% phenol and 1.1% croton oil. **b**) The patient 1 year later. (Reprinted from Plastic Surgery 2/e, Mathes SJ, chapter: Face Lift (Lower Face): Current Techniques by Fardo D, Zins JE, Nahai F, ©2005 Elsevier Inc. With permission from Elsevier.)

tical Corp.; Hylaform, Inamed Corp.) has replaced collagen compounds as the most popular filler. According to the American Society for Aesthetic Plastic Surgery, hyaluronic acid injections have become the fifth most-common nonsurgical cosmetic procedure, after botulinum toxin A, laser hair removal, microdermabrasion, and chemical peeling techniques. Approximately 880,000 hyaluronic acid injections were performed by board-certified plastic surgeons, otolaryngologists, and dermatologists in 2004, according to Society statistics.[53]

Common areas for hyaluronic acid injections include the nasolabial folds, the triangle between the alar base and the nasolabial folds, the commissure, and the upper and lower lips. Generally, botulinum toxin A is preferable for the upper face and Restylane for the lower face.

Finally, skin quality can be improved in concert with the above procedures. Resurfacing can be accomplished with CO_2 laser resurfacing, Erbium laser resurfacing, or phenol-croton oil peeling techniques.[54-61] All resurfacing techniques carry

the risk of hypopigmentation because all reduce the melanocyte population if taken into the intermediate dermis or deeper. If vertical rhytids of the upper and lower lips are to be adequately treated, the injury needs to extend to this level. Therefore, ideal candidates for deep resurfacing techniques are light-skinned individuals.

All three of the above modalities effectively treat vertical rhytids. In our experience, phenol-croton oil peeling is the most effective, followed by CO_2 laser resurfacing and Erbium laser resurfacing in ablation of vertical rhytids (Figure 9-6). Recent articles by Hetter and by Stone and Lefer discuss phenol-croton oil peeling in depth.[57-61]

The Neck

The standard operation for correcting lower facial aging remains the cervicofacial rhytidectomy, but lesser approaches have increasing appeal.

Over the past 25 years, surgeons have noted the increased ability of neck skin to contract

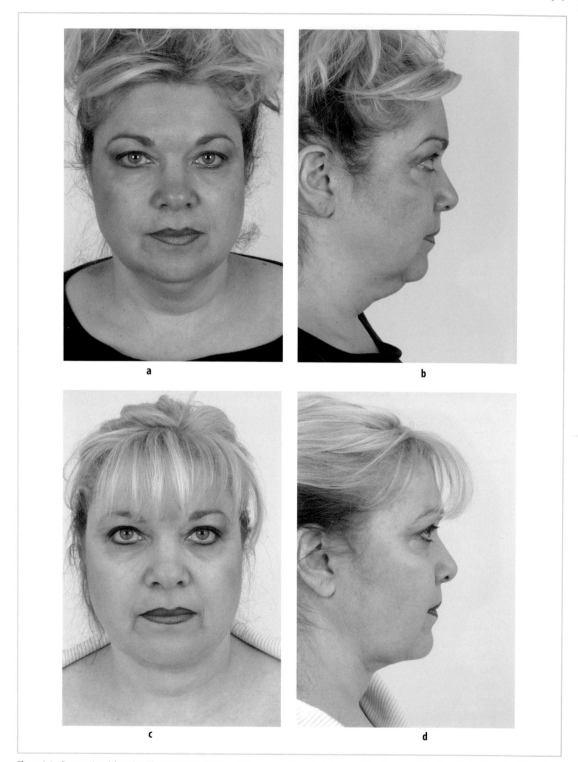

Figure 9-9. Preoperative **a**) frontal and **b**) lateral view of a 50-year old woman with substantial submental and submandibular fat and mild skin laxity. **c**) Frontal and **d**) lateral view of the patient 6 months after anterior lipectomy and platysmaplasty.

The operation is technically easy to perform, and complications are few. As mentioned, over-resection of fat should be avoided as this will lead to skeletization of neck, visibility of the platysmal muscle attached to skin, and other irregularities. Marginal mandibular neuropraxia is reasonably common and invariably resolves within 2 weeks. No hematomas have occurred in our last 50 procedures.

Patients with a marked amount of skin excess and poor skin elasticity are generally not good candidates for this procedure because their skin will not adequately contract once undermined. These patients are better treated by either standard cervicofacial rhytidectomy or by direct neck excision platysmaplasty through an anterior approach and Z-plasty.[74] In fact, men in their mid-70s and 80s are ideal patients for direct neck skin excision. The results with direct neck skin excision will be superior to those of cervicofacial rhytidectomy because, once again, skin excision is being performed directly over the area where skin excess and laxity are the greatest. These patients invariably have residual excess skin if cervicofacial rhytidectomy is performed. Further, given these patients' age, this operation is quicker, safer, and the scars tend to be nonproblematic (Figures 9-10a, 9-10b, 9-10c, and 9-10d).

Postbariatric Surgery

Given the epidemic of obesity that has afflicted Americans, gastric bypass surgery—its multiple variations known collectively as bariatric surgery—has become increasingly popular. More than 103,000 bariatric surgical procedures were performed in 2003.[75]

Between 15% and 20% of patients undergoing bariatric surgery eventually seek plastic surgery once their weight has stabilized. A patient's weight must usually be stable for 1 year before plastic surgery is considered to correct skin excess. Potential areas and procedures include the abdomen, the thighs, the hips, arms, and face and neck. Each patient may require multiple operations to treat multiple areas, and the estimated number of these operations is substantial.

Patients seeking facial rejuvenation after massive weight loss present with many problems similar to those of other facial rejuvenation patients, but they also have some unique problems. Massive-weight-loss patients tend to have substantially more excess facial and neck skin. They also may have soft tissue atrophy in the submalar areas and deeper nasolabial folds than do patients who present with facial aging only. Therefore, in addition to cervicofacial rhytidectomy, other procedures may also be required at the same time or in the future.

A common first-step in these patients includes a face and neck lift and platysmaplasty. Skin incisions should be altered with the realization that a large amount of excess skin will be excised. Therefore, both the temporal and the post-auricular hairline should be preserved. Hair-bearing skin should not be excised. A horizontal cut along the sideburn-cheek junction anteriorly with a vertical incision extending just posterior to the anterior hairline is the desired anterior incision.[76] Posteriorly, the postauricular incision should follow the posterior hairline at the neck-hairline junction. Further posteriorly, the incision should extend into the hair-bearing scalp. Because of the large amount of excess skin that may be present in the submental area, the patient should be warned that some excess skin may recur in this area and may even require secondary correction.

Marked soft tissue atrophy in the submalar area may be an indication for placing submalar Silastic implants at the time of face and neck lift. We prefer this technique for treating soft tissue atrophy in this area. The submalar implants tends to provide permanent augmentation, do not resorb, and avoid the difficulty of harvesting fat in a patient who has already undergone massive weight loss.

Secondary surgery, in women as well as men, may include a direct excision in the area of the nasolabial folds because of their marked depth (Figure 9-11).

In summary, the patient undergoing facelift surgery after massive weight loss may require not only cervicofacial rhytidectomy but implant augmentation in cases of severe soft tissue atrophy. Secondary procedures, including revision neck lift and excision of the nasolabial folds, may also be in order.

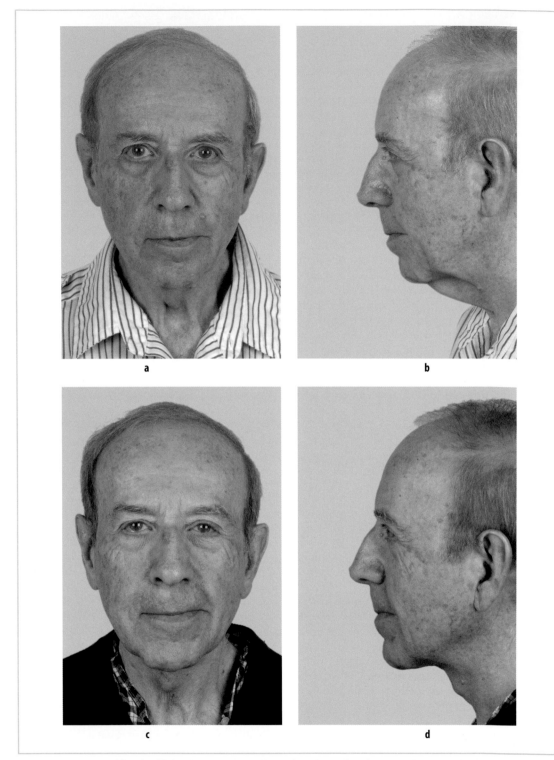

Figure 9-10. Preoperative **a**) frontal and **b**) lateral view of a 76-year-old man who underwent direct skin excision of the neck with Z-plasty and platysmaplasty. **c**) Frontal and **d**) lateral view of the patient 6 months after anterior lipectomy and platysmaplasty.

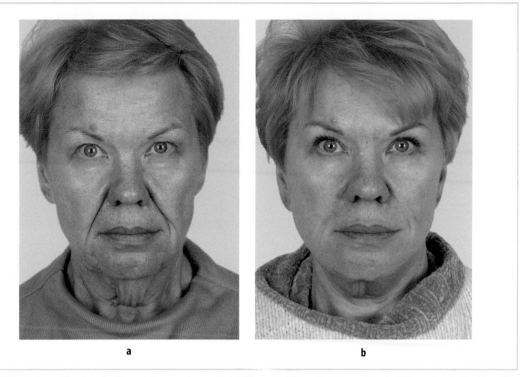

Figure 9-11. a) Preoperative view of a 58-year-old woman who recently lost 110 pounds. **b**) The patient 1 year after a facelift, secondary direct excision of the nasolabial folds, and CO_2 laser resurfacing of the scars. (Reprinted from Plastic Surgery 2/e, Mathes SJ, chapter: Face Lift (Lower Face): Current Techniques by Fardo D, Zins JE, Nahai F, ©2005 Elsevier Inc. With permission from Elsevier.)

Correcting Lipodystrophy in HIV/AIDS Patients

Just as bariatric surgery has increased the number of patients seeking plastic surgery after massive weight loss, successful treatment of patients with HIV/AIDS has increased the number of requests for surgery in this patient population.[77,78] Highly aggressive antiretroviral therapy is prolonging remissions in these patients but has also led to a clear lipodystrophy syndrome characterized by central obesity and peripheral soft tissue atrophy.

Specifically, these patients display facial-wasting syndrome, which is characterized by a loss of submalar soft tissue that increases the depth of the nasolabial fold and that exaggerates the prominence of the zygoma. This degree of facial wasting is variable and is graded 1 to 4, 1 being the most mild and 4 the most severe.[79]

This syndrome has been recognized only since 1998, so few reports of surgical treatment for these patients have been published, and no large series is available. The approach to these patients is not straightforward. They may have submental and submandibular lipodystrophy. However, this lipodystrophy tends to be less fatty, more fibrous, and not easily amenable to routine liposuction. Therefore, ultrasound-assisted liposuction is more efficacious and is recommended (Figure 9-12).

Facial atrophy, as described above, has been treated with fat injections, dermis fat grafts, and Silastic submalar implants.[80–83] The studies cited above are small retrospective patient series with short follow-ups; thus, outcomes data are currently weak.

Conceptually, fat injections to recipient areas of soft tissue atrophy are problematic. The short-term results of the above studies do not contradict this notion. Finally, submalar implant

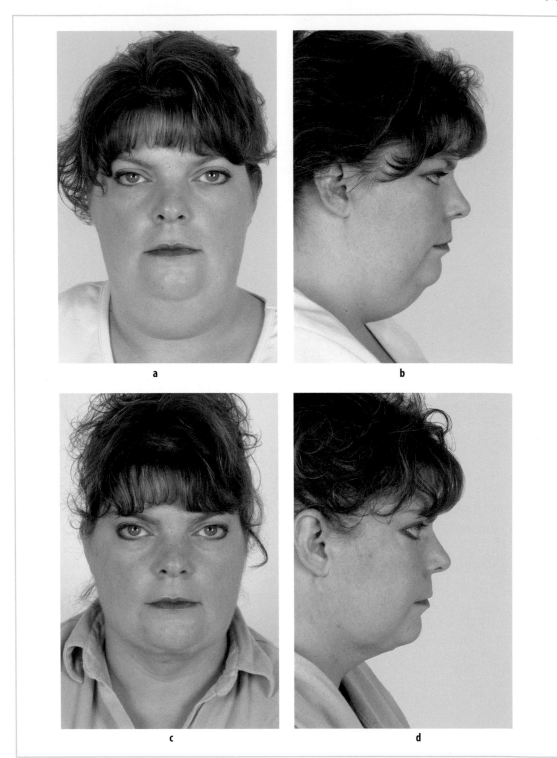

Figure 9-12. Preoperative **a**) frontal and **b**) lateral view of a 35-year-old [[man/woman]] with HIV-associated lipodystrophy characterized by submental and subman-dibular fat excess and peripheral wasting after highly aggressive antiretroviral therapy (HAART). **c**) Frontal and **d**) lateral view of the patient 6 months later.

augmentation, in the absence of infection and extrusion, has potential for long-term success. Therefore, we employ submental and submandibular liposuction using ultrasound-assisted techniques for submental lipodystrophy and the obtuse cervicomental angle and Silastic submalar implant augmentation to repair submalar soft tissue atrophy.

Conclusion

In conclusion, endoscopic and minimally invasive techniques are receiving increasing interest from patients and the media. The endoscopic browlift, endoscopically assisted midface or open mid-face correction, rejuvenation of the perioral area, and anterior-only approaches to the neck and the results have been illustrated here. Plastic surgery after massive weight loss will become increasingly common over the next several years. A logical approach to treating these patients is also described. Finally, because of improved survival with newer treatments for HIV, patients with lipodystrophy after AIDS treatment will increasingly seek plastic surgery correction. The plastic surgeon is well advised to be prepared to treat these new patient populations.

References

1. Core GB, Vasconez LO, Graham HD III. Endoscopic browlift. *Clin Plast Surg.* 1995;22:619–631.
2. Oslin B, Core GB, Vasconez LO. The biplanar endoscopically assisted forehead lift. *Clin Plast Surg.* 1995;22:633–638.
3. Ramirez OM. Endoscopically assisted biplanar forehead lift. *Plast Reconstr Surg.* 1995;96:323–333.
4. Ramirez OM. The anchor subperiosteal forehead lift. *Plast Reconstr Surg.* 1995;95:993–1003.
5. Moody FP, Losken A, Bostwick J 3rd, Trinei FA, Eaves FF III. Endoscopic frontal branch neurectomy, corrugator myectomy, and brow lift for forehead asymmetry after facial nerve palsy. *Plast Reconstr Surg.* 2001;108:218–223.
6. Gruber RP, Nahai F. Brow or forehead fixation with sutures only: a preliminary communication. *Aesthetic Plast Surg.* 2003;27:403–405.
7. Eaves FF 3rd, Bostwick J 3rd, Nahai F. Instrumentation and setup for endoscopic plastic surgery. *Clin Plast Surg.* 1995;22:591–603.
8. Byrd HS, Burt JD. Achieving aesthetic balance in the brow, eyelids, and midface. *Plast Reconstr Surg.* 2002;110:926–33; discussion 934–939.
9. Byrd HS. The extended browlift. *Clin Plast Surg.* 1997;24:233–246.
10. Hunt JA, Byrd HS. The deep temporal lift: a multiplanar lateral brow, temporal, and upper face lift. *Plast Reconstr Surg.* 2002;110:1793–1796.
11. de la Fuente A, Honig JF. Video-assisted endoscopic transtemporal multilayer upper midface lift MUM-Lift). *J Craniofac Surg.* 2005;16:267–276.
12. De Cordier BC, de la Torre JI, Al-Hakeem MS, Rosenberg LZ, Gardner PM, Costa-Ferreira A, et al. Endoscopic forehead lift: review of technique, cases, and complications. *Plast Reconstr Surg.* 2002;110:1558–1568; discussion 1569–1570.
13. Stuzin JM, Baker TJ, Baker TM. Anchor subperiosteal forehead lift: from open to endoscopic. *Plast Reconstr Surg.* 2001;107:872–873.
14. Ramirez OM. Anchor subperiosteal forehead lift: from open to endoscopic. *Plast Reconstr Surg.* 2001;107:868–871.
15. Landecker A, Buck JB, Grotting JC. A new resorbable tack fixation technique for endoscopic brow lifts. *Plast Reconstr Surg.* 2003;111:880–886.
16. Evans GR, Kelishadi SS, Ho KU for the Plastic Surgery Educational Foundation DATA Committee. "Heads up" on brow lift with Coapt Systems' Endotine Forehead technology. *Plast Reconstr Surg.* 2004;113:1504–1505.
17. Holzapfel AM, Mangat DS. Endoscopic forehead-lift using a bioabsorbable fixation device. *Arch Facial Plast Surg.* 2004;6:389–393.
18. Guyuron B, Behmand RA, Green R. Shortening of the long forehead. *Plast Reconstr Surg.* 1999;103:218–223.
19. Gonzalez AM, Papay F, Zins JE. Calvarial thickness and its relation to cranial bone harvest. *Plast Reconstr Surg.* In press.
20. Hamra ST. Prevention and correction of the "face-lifted" appearance. *Facial Plast Surg.* 2000;16:215–229.
21. Hamra ST. The zygorbicular dissection in composite rhytidectomy: an ideal midface plane. *Plast Reconstr Surg.* 1998;102:1646–1657.
22. Hamra ST. Arcus marginalis release and orbital fat preservation in midface rejuvenation. *Plast Reconstr Surg.* 1995;96:354–362.
23. Hamra ST. Composite rhytidectomy and the nasolabial fold. *Clin Plast Surg.* 1995;22:313–324.
24. Connell BF, Marten TJ. The trifurcated SMAS flap: three-part segmentation of the conventional flap for improved results in the midface, cheek, and neck. *Aesthetic Plast Surg.* 1995;19:415–420.
25. Owsley JQ Jr, Zweifler M. Midface lift of the malar fat pad: technical advances. *Plast Reconstr Surg.* 2002;110:674–685.
26. Owsley JQ. Rejuvenation of the midface. *Plast Reconstr Surg.* 2001;108:262.
27. Owsley JQ. Elevation of the malar fat pad superficial to the orbicularis oculi muscle for correction of prominent nasolabial folds. *Clin Plast Surg.* 1995;22:279–293.
28. Stuzin JM, Baker TJ, Baker TM. Refinements in face lifting: enhanced facial contour using Vicryl mesh incorporated into SMAS fixation. *Plast Reconstr Surg.* 2000;105:290–301.
29. Stuzin JM, Baker TJ, Gordon HL, Baker TM. Extended SMAS dissection as an approach to midface rejuvenation. *Clin Plast Surg.* 1995;22:295–311.
30. Ramirez OM. The central oval of the face: tridimensional endoscopic rejuvenation. *Facial Plast Surg.* 2000;16:283–298.
31. Ramirez OM. Three-dimensional endoscopic midface enhancement: a personal quest for the ideal cheek

rejuvenation. Plast Reconstr Surg. 2002;109:329–340; discussion 341–349.

32. Ramirez OM. Treatment of the aging midface. Plast Reconstr Surg. 2000;106:1653–1656.

33. Ramirez OM. Endoscopic full facelift. Aesthetic Plast Surg. 1994;18:363.

34. Little JW. Three-dimensional rejuvenation of the midface: volumetric resculpture by malar imbrication. Plast Reconstr Surg. 2000;105:267–285.

35. Little JW. Volumetric perceptions in midfacial aging with altered priorities for rejuvenation. Plast Reconstr Surg. 2000;105:252–266.

36. de la Torre JI, Rosenberg LZ, De Cordier BC, Gardner PM, Fix RJ, Vasconez LO. Clinical analysis of malar fat pad re-elevation. Ann Plast Surg. 2003;50:244–248.

37. De Cordier BC, de la Torre JI, Al-Hakeem MS, Rosenberg LZ, Costa-Ferreira A, Gardner PM, et al. Rejuvenation of the midface by elevating the malar fat pad: review of technique, cases, and complications. Plast Reconstr Surg. 2002;110:1526–1536.

38. Seify H, Jones G, Bostwick J, Hester TR. Endoscopic-assisted face lift: review of 200 cases. Ann Plast Surg. 2004;52:234–239.

39. Hester TR Jr, Codner MA, McCord CD, Nahai F, Giannopoulos A. Evolution of technique of the direct transblepharoplasty approach for the correction of lower lid and midfacial aging: maximizing results and minimizing complications in a 5-year experience. Plast Reconstr Surg. 2000;105:393–406; discussion 407–408.

40. Tonnard PL, Verpaele AM. The MACS-Lift Short-Scar Rhytidectomy. St. Louis: Quality Medical Publishing Inc, 2004.

41. Wu W. Sutures in facial rejuvenation. Aesth Surg J. 2004;24:582.

42. Aiache A. Rejuvenation of the perioral area. Dermatol Clin. 1997;15:665–672.

43. Austin HW. The lip lift. Plast Reconstr Surg.1986;77:990–994.

44. Austin HW, Weston GW. Rejuvenation of the aging mouth. Clin Plast Surg. 1992;19:511–524.

45. Fanous N. Correction of thin lips: lip lift. Plast Reconstr Surg. 1984;74:33.

46. Feldman G. Direct upper lip lifting: a safe procedure. Aesth Plast Surg. 1993;17:291.

47. Greenwald AE. The lip lift: cheiloplasty for cheiloptosis. Am J Cosm Surg. 1985;2:16.

48. Sigal RK, Poindexter B, Weston GW, et al. Rejuvenating the aged face. Perspect Outlook Plast Surg. 2000;14:1.

49. Lassus C. Surgical vermilion augmentation: different possibilities. Aesth Plast Surg. 1992;16:123.

50. Rozner L, Isaacs GW. Lip lifting. Br J Plast Surg. 1981;34:481–484.

51. Coleman SR. Facial recontouring with lipostructure. Clin Plast Surg. 1997;24:347–367.

52. Coleman SR. Structural fat grafts: the ideal filler? Clin Plast Surg. 2001;28:111–119.

53. The American Society for Aesthetic Plastic Surgery, Cosmetic Surgery National Data Bank Statistics, 2004.

54. Weinstein C, Roberts TL. Aesthetic skin resurfacing with the high-energy Ultrapulse CO_2 laser. Clin Plast Surg. 1997;24:379.

55. Pozner JN, Roberts TL. Variable-pulse width ER: YAG laser resurfacing. Clin Plast Surg. 2000;27:263.

56. Stuzin JM. Phenol peeling and the history of phenol peeling. Clin Plast Surg. 1998;25:1.

57. Hetter GP. An examination of the phenol-croton oil peel, part IV: face peel results with different concentrations of phenol and croton oil. Plast Reconstr Surg. 2000;105:1061–1083; discussion 1084–1087.

58. Hetter GP. An examination of the phenol-croton oil peel, part III: the plastic surgeon's role. Plast Reconstr Surg. 2000;105:752–763.

59. Hetter GP. An examination of the phenol-croton oil peel, part II: the lay peelers and their croton oil formulas. Plast Reconstr Surg. 2000;105:240–248; discussion 249–251.

60. Hetter GP. An examination of the phenol-croton oil peel, part I: dissecting the formula. Plast Reconstr Surg. 2000;105:227–239; discussion 249–251.

61. Stone PA, Lefer LG. Modified phenol chemical face peels: recognizing the role of application techniques. Clin Plast Surg. 2001;28:13.

62. Courtiss EH. Suction lipectomy of the neck. Plast Reconstr Surg. 1985;76:882.

63. Goddio AS. Skin retraction following suction lipectomy by treatment site: a study of 500 procedures in 458 selected subjects. Plast Reconstr Surg. 1991;87:66.

64. Giampapa VC, DiBernardo BE. Neck recontouring with suture suspension and liposuction: an alternative for early rhytidectomy candidate. Aesth Plast Surg. 1995;19:217.

65. Giampapa VC. Suture suspension offers predictable long-lasting neck rejuvenation. Aesth Surg Journ. 2000;20:253.

66. Robbins LB, Shaw KE. En bloc cervical lipectomy for treatment of the problem neck in facial rejuvenation surgery. Plast Reconstr Surg. 1989;83:53–60.

67. Feldman JJ. My Approach to Face-Neck-Brow-Periorbital Lift. Instructional Course 409 for the American Society of Plastic Surgeons annual meeting, San Antonio, TX, November 2002.

68. Feldman JJ. The Isolated Neck Lift. Massachusetts General Hospital Aesthetic Symposium, Vail, CO, March 1996.

69. Feldman JJ. Face or neck lift without a post auricular incision. 33rd Annual Meeting of the American Society of Aesthetic Surgery, Orlando, FL, May 2000.

70. Feldman JJ. Small Incision Necklift. Instructional Course 408 for the American Society of Aesthetic Surgery annual meetng, Vancouver, Canada, April 2004.

71. Knize DM. Limited incision submental lipectomy and platysmaplasty. Plast Reconstr Surg. 2004;113:1275–1278.

72. Knize DM. Limited incision submental lipectomy and platysmaplasty. Plast Reconstr Surg. 1998;101:473–481.

73. Zins JE, Fardo D. The "anterior-only" approach to neck rejuvenation: an alternative to facelift surgery. Plast Reconstr Surg. In press.

74. Gradinger GP. Anterior cervicoplasty in the male patient. Plast Reconstr Surg. 2000;106:1146.

75. Kazel R. Insurers trim bariatric surgery coverage. AMNews.com. Accessed April 2004.

76. Guyuron B, Watkins F, Totonchi A. Modified temporal incision for facial rhytidectomy: an 18-year experience. Plast Reconstr Surg. 2005;115:609–616.

77. Strauch B, Baum T, Robbins N. Treatment of human immunodeficiency virus-associated lipodystrophy with dermafat graft transfer to the malar area. Plast Reconstr Surg. 2004;113:363–370; discussion 371–372.

78. Talmor M, Hoffman LA, LaTrenta GS. Facial atrophy in HIV-related fat redistribution syndrome: anatomic evaluation and surgical reconstruction. *Ann Plast Surg.* 2002;49:11–17; discussion 117–118.

79. James J, Carruthers A, Carruthers J. HIV-associated facial lipoatrophy. *Dermatol Surg.* 2002;28:979–986.

80. Gooderham M, Solish N. Use of hyaluronic acid for soft tissue augmentation of HIV-associated facial lipodystrophy. *Dermatol Surg.* 2005;31:104–108.

81. Valantin MA, Aubron-Olivier C, Ghosn J, Laglenne E, Pauchard M, Schoen H, et al. Polylactic acid implants (New-Fill) to correct facial lipoatrophy in HIV-infected patients: results of the open-label study VEGA. *AIDS.* 2003;17:2471–2477.

82. Levan P, Nguyen TH, Lallemand F, Mazetier L, Mimoun M, Rozenbaum W, et al. Correction of facial lipoatrophy in HIV-infected patients on highly active antiretroviral therapy by injection of autologous fatty tissue. *AIDS.* 2002;16:1985–1987.

83. Serra-Renom JM, Fontdevila J. Treatment of facial fat atrophy related to treatment with protease inhibitors by autologous fat injection in patients with human immunodeficiency virus infection. *Plast Reconstr Surg.* 2004;114:551–555; discussion 556–557.

10

Perspectives for Facial Allograft Transplantation in Humans

Maria Z. Siemionow and Galip Agaoglu

Introduction

The face is a functional as well as an esthetic part of the body. It is the window through which we interact with others: two thirds of our communication is through nonverbal facial expressions. Reconstructing partial or full facial deformities caused by burns, trauma, or tumors still challenges most reconstructive surgeons. The ideal reconstructive procedure should address both the functional and esthetic units of the face.

Conventional Reconstructive Methods

Conventional methods for reconstructing facial deformities include skin grafts, local and distant flaps, prefabricated flaps, expanded flaps, and free flaps. The success of these methods varies.

Successful results have been obtained after total face resurfacing using monoblock full-thickness skin grafts.[1,2] Although color and texture matches are reasonably satisfactory in the short term, the long-term follow-up is usually associated with skin graft contractures and color changes that result in an unsatisfactory final outcome.

Since the introduction of prefabricated flaps in reconstructing facial subunits,[3] satisfactory results have been reported with prefabrication and expansion of the nearby normal tissues.[4,5] Axial pattern flaps, prefabricated from the supraclavicular skin using antebrachial fascia based on the radial vessels, have been used to reconstruct the entire face after sever burns.[6] Unfortunately, in facial burns, the adjacent skin is also partially or completely involved, making adequate reconstruction almost impossible.

Tissue expanders have been applied to expand the adjacent skin to achieve sufficient tissue of identical color and texture for facial reconstruction[7-9] Tissue expanders can also be used to create full-thickness skin grafts for complete or partial resurfacing of the face.[10] As with prefabricated flaps however, adjacent skin may be involved in the injury, which may prohibit the use of tissue expanders. Other potential problems relate to the choice of expander, the site of insertion of the expander, the elevation and suturing of the expanded flap, and the management of the free margins of the flaps.[9]

The first free-tissue transfer was performed to reconstruct burn deformities.[11] This innovation led to enormous advances in reconstructive microsurgery, and different types of free tissues were transferred from distant parts of the body to reconstruct facial deformities. The facial subunit approach, introduced by Burget, was based on modifying the recipient defect and donor tissue.[12] Feldman introduced "the single sheet concept" in resurfacing of the whole face after facial burns.[13] This concept led to a bilateral, extended scapular-parascapular free flap, incorporating bilateral superficial circumflex scapular vessels, that was used for total face resurfacing in patients with severe facial burns with good-to-fair results.[14] Although various types of free flaps have been used for reconstructing the face, the functional and aesthetic outcome have not been optimum.

Miller et al. reported the first successful replantation of the entire scalp.[15] Thereafter, replantations of many cases of partial or complete scalp avulsions were reported, including forehead, ear, eyebrow, and eyelid, with abundant regrowth of hair and return of scalp sensibility.[16] Successful replantation of different avulsed segments of the face, including the nose, ear, and upper and lower lips, also reported.[17-19]

Although many cases of scalp and face-segment replantation have been reported worldwide, only two successful cases of total face and scalp replantation have been reported.[20,21] In the first, replantation was performed in 2 pieces, based on the medial canthal vein and the facial vein and artery on the right side and the labial artery with its vein and superficial temporal artery and two concomitant veins on the left side. Three years after replantation, the patient recovered satisfactory animation of the oral musculature and profound growth of hair on the scalp.[20] In the second case, the face was avulsed as one piece, including the entire scalp, right ear, forehead, eyebrows, right cheek, nose, and upper lip. This replantation was based only on single superficial temporal artery and two veins. Four months postoperatively, the patient had hair growth and normal mimetic function.[21] Because the optimal outcome was obtained after replanting the avulsed segments of the face and scalp, every effort should be made to achieve successful replantation, even if the avulsed scalp and face contain several lacerations and contusions.

Although many techniques have been described for reconstructing severe facial injuries, total resurfacing of the face with a single soft, pliable tissue, matched in color and texture, is almost impossible. There is simply no such tissue in the body that is of similar quality that gives the characteristics of a normal face. The final outcome after all these conventional reconstructive procedures is far from ideal because they result in a tight, mask-like face with lack of facial expression and an unsatisfactory cosmetic appearance. Recent advances in composite tissue allograft transplantation have initiated a new period in the field of reconstructive surgery.

Clinical Applications of Composite Tissue Allografts

The aspiration of surgeons for tissue transplantation dates back to the third century AD, when the sainted twins Cosmas and Damian amputated a gangrenous leg of a Roman patient and replaced it with a limb taken from a dead Moor.[22] Advances in the field of reconstructive surgery made the feasibility of composite tissue allograft (CTA) transplantation a clinical reality. CTA transplants have been performed to improve, rather than to save, the quality of life of patients with disabilities. Since the first successful hand transplantation in 1998, more than 50 CTA transplants have been carried out worldwide including 25 hands, 9 abdominal wall transplants, 8 knees, 7 nerve allografts, 2 flexor tendon apparatus, 1 larynx, 1 skeletal muscle, and 1 tongue transplant.[23-35]

The ultimate goal for CTA transplantation is the induction of donor-specific tolerance without the need for chronic immunosuppression. Different strategies for tolerance induction have been developed in experimental studies, including: costimulation blockade by using different monoclonal antibodies, immunoablation with hematologic reconstitution and allogeneic mixed chimerism.[36-38]

Currently, bone marrow transplantation is the only clinical way to achieve tolerance by inducing mixed hematopoietic chimerism. This tolerance was first noticed in a patient with multiple myeloma who underwent bone marrow and renal transplantation after conditioning with a nonmyeloablative protocol of cyclophosphamide, antithymocyte globulin, and thymic irradiation. The patient was treated only with cyclosporine A for 73 days after transplant and the kidney was accepted without chronic immunosuppressive therapy.[39]

Simultaneous bone marrow and renal transplantation is being performed in Boston without long-term immunosuppression. So far, all the grafts have been accepted.[28] Although clinical tolerance has been proven in these patients, they needed toxic preconditioning before bone marrow transplantation, which cannot be done with composite tissue allografts.

Facial Allograft Transplantation

Facial transplantation is the next step in CTA transplantation to treat patients whose facial disfigurement cannot be addressed by conventional methods of reconstructive surgery.

The only successful scalp transplantation was performed between identical twins.[40] A woman had 50% to 60% of her scalp avulsed. Initial coverage with split-thickness skin grafts and subsequent multiple punch grafts from her identical twin were performed with moderate success. The twins were HLA identical and had identical blood groups. Mixed lymphocyte reaction was nonreactive. From her identical twin, the patient received 2 free scalp flaps measuring 19 cm × 3.5 cm and 17 cm × 3 cm, respectively, in two sessions. The flaps were based on superficial temporal arteries. At 6 months follow-up, without any immunosuppressive regimen, the flaps provided adequate hair growth.

It is difficult to anticipate the look of a face after transplantation because patients with severe facial disfigurement undergo multiple reconstructive procedures. However, computer studies suggest that the face would display more of the characteristics of the recipient skeleton than of the donor soft tissues.[41]

Skin, as a component of CTA, is considered to be the most antigenic tissue of the body. A vascularized skin allograft, unlike nonvascularized skin allograft, is a good source for dendritic cells, which migrate from the donor to the recipient through hematogenous and lymphatic systems. These cells are important in allograft acceptance.

Over the past 15 years, we have focused on methods to induce tolerance for composite tissue transplants. We used different models of highly antigenic CTA transplants (hind limb, full face, hemiface and groin skin flap models), including skin, as a component of these transplants, for tolerance induction.[42-53]

Reconstructive surgeons attempting to transplant facial allografts must address several technical feasibility and applicability issues, develop protocols for lifelong immunosuppression, and resolve the associated ethical, social, and psychological concerns. Other issues that also need to be addressed are obtaining Institutional Review Board approval, identifying appropriate recipients thorough screening for inclusion and exclusion criteria, and finding appropriate donors.

Technical Feasibility and Applicability

The outcome of conventional reconstructive procedures is unsatisfactory because most of the tissues used do not have the quality and characteristics of the face. According to Gillies principle of "replacing like with like," the only remaining option for obtaining optimal functional and aesthetic results is facial allograft transplantation. Although facial transplantation has not yet been performed, 2 successful cases of total face and scalp replantation have been reported with excellent outcomes.[20,21]

Experimental studies on hemifacial and full-facial transplantation in dog and rodent models have been performed with success. Our cadaveric study revealed that after injection, methylene blue dye perfused to skin and dermal plexuses of the flap and was well visualized from the external carotid artery up to the terminal branches of the facial and superficial temporal arteries.

The vascular anatomy of the human face is well known. There are rich vascular plexuses in the subcutaneous tissue. The face is bilaterally supplied by the branches of the external carotid arteries, mainly the facial and superficial temporal arteries, and it is drained by the external jugular and facial veins. An entire facial skin flap, based on the facial and superficial temporal arteries, could be transplanted. Different components of the facial tissues can be incorporated in this flap, including skin, facial expression muscles, the facial nerve, and bones. Initially, not to further complicate this already complicated procedure; only skin should be transplanted to the face. Once facial skin flap transplantation is successful, other components of the face can be considered.

One of the crucial issues that should be considered when planning facial transplantation, as with any microsurgical procedure, is the risk of failure of the vascular anastomoses. Vascular failure, diagnosed in the early stages of transplantation, can be treated by exploring the vascular pedicles and redoing the anastomoses. If all attempts to salvage the flap fail, the rescue procedure should be planned and defect should be covered with vascularized skin flaps or autologous skin grafts.

Experimental, Vascularized Nonfacial Skin Allografts

Hind Limb Allograft Transplant Model

We have shown that stable donor-specific multilineage chimerism is associated with induction of tolerance in the hind limb allografts, where the skin component of the transplant was vascularized.

Experimental Model. Limb transplants across major histocompatibility (MHC) barriers were performed between fully allogeneic BN (RT1^n)

and semiallogeneic LBN (RT1^{1+n}) donors and Lewis recipients (LEW; RT1^l).[42–46]

Immunosuppressive Protocol. Different immuno-suppressive protocols of CsA alone, combined CsA with $\alpha\beta$-TCR monoclonal antibody ($\alpha\beta$-TCRmAb), and combined CsA-anti-lymphocyte serum (ALS) for different periods of time were used. The efficiency of immunosuppressive protocols and donor-specific chimerism was assessed by flow cytometry. Clinical tolerance and immunocompetence were confirmed by skin grafting in vivo and by mixed lymphocyte reaction in vitro. Combined protocols of Cs-/$\alpha\beta$-TCRmAb, and CsA-ALS resulted in long-term survival and donor-specific tolerance.

Limb allografts differ from composite facial allografts because they have a bone marrow element, which may be essential in inducing tolerance.

Vascularized Skin (Groin) Allograft Transplant Model

A vascularized skin allograft transplant model was used to evaluate the potential for tolerance induction in highly immunogenic tissue grafts (e.g., skin). We tested the efficacy of different immunosuppressive protocols and their potential to extend survival and to induce chimerism in vascularized skin allografts.

Experimental Model. Vascularized skin allograft transplants across strong MHC barriers were performed between fully allogeneic ACI (RT1^a) donors and LEW (RT1^l) recipients.[52] Skin flaps (3 × 4 cm), based on the femoral artery and vein, were harvested from the donor groin and included the underlying panniculus carnosus and inguinal fat tissue. In the recipient animal, a defect of the same size was created on the right side, and artery and vein were anastomosed end-to-end with the recipient's femoral artery and vein.

Immunosuppressive Protocol. Vascularized skin allograft transplants were treated with different immunosuppressive protocols. The animals received $\alpha\beta$-TCRmAb, CsA, or FK506 monotherapy or a combination of $\alpha\beta$-TCRmAb-CsA and $\alpha\beta$-TCRmAb-FK506. Immunosuppressive therapy started at the day of transplantation and continued for 7 days. The combined $\alpha\beta$-TCRmAb-CsA and $\alpha\beta$-TCRmAb-FK506 protocols were effective in inducing and maintaining chimerism and substantially extended the survival of the vascularized skin allograft transplants.

These strategies can be applied to other CTA and solid organ transplants. Furthers studies on dosage modification and augmentation of chimerism with bone marrow transplantation are currently underway.

Experimental Facial Allograft Transplantations

A Canine Model of Hemifacial Transplant

Experimental Model. A hemifacial transplant between 2 dogs was performed to determine the viability of a facial transplant using facial artery and external jugular vein as pedicles.[54] A skin muscle flap in the superficial musculoaponeurotic system plane based on the facial artery and external jugular vein was harvested. In the recipient animal, the artery and vein were anastomosed to the lingual artery and external jugular vein, respectively.

Immunosuppressive Protocol. Cyclosporine A (4 mg/kg/day) and prednisone (1 mg/kg/day) were given for immunosuppression. The flap was rejected by day 6, and the dog was euthanized. This study was anatomical and not a test of an immunological transplant model.

Composite Full Facial-Scalp Transplant Model

We attempted to determine the best option for reconstructing the face and scalp; with the rationale that allogeneic transplantation would provide the best aesthetic and functional results. On the basis of our 15 years' experience with composite allograft transplantations, we introduced a composite full-facial and scalp transplantation model in rats to evaluate its technical feasibility, immunological aspects, and potential for future clinical applications.

Experimental Model. Composite total facial and scalp allograft transplants were performed between Lewis-Brown Norway (LBN RT1) donors and Lewis (LEW, RT1) recipients.[49,50] The full-facial–scalp flap was harvested as a single unit based on the bilateral common carotid arteries and the external jugular veins and included the entire facial skin, scalp, and external ears. In the recipients, the facial skin and scalp, including the external ear, were excised as a full-thickness skin graft in which the facial nerve and muscles were preserved. The periorbital and perioral regions were also preserved to prevent functional deficiencies, which could impair feeding or breathing (Figure 10-1). Either the common or external carotid arteries and the anterior facial veins were used for anastomoses.

Immunosuppressive Protocol. The animals received CsA monotherapy (16 mg/kg/day) without recipient preconditioning. Therapy was begun the day of surgery, tapered to 2 mg/kg/day over 4 weeks, and then continued at this dose until the end of the study. The flaps survived 200 days. This study confirmed the feasibility and applicability of the total facial and scalp allograft transplantation across major histocompatibility barriers and was the first to confirm long-term survival of full-facial allograft transplants under low maintenance doses of CsA monotherapy in a rat model (Figure 10-2).

A New Surgical Approach for Full-Facial–Scalp Transplant

To improve survival, we modified the arterial anastomoses in these full-facial–scalp allograft transplants.

Experimental Model. Full-facial–scalp allograft transplants were done across MHC barriers between fully allogeneic ACI (RT1[a]) donor rats and Lewis (RT1) recipient rats.[53] The composite facial-scalp flap, including the external ear component, was harvested as described and was based on bilateral common carotid arteries and external jugular veins. In the recipient, the facial skin and scalp, including the external ears, were excised as a full-thickness graft. In all transplants, veins were anastomosed to the external jugular vein or to the posterior facial vein on the left side and to anterior facial vein on the right side.

The arterial anastomoses in the recipients were modified as follows. After anastomosing the left common carotid artery of the flap to the left common carotid artery of the recipient end-to-side, the right common carotid artery of the flap was anastomosed either to the left common carotid artery of the flap, end-to-side, or end-to-end to the stump of the internal carotid artery on the left side of the flap, which was kept long during harvesting.

Immunosuppressive Protocol. All the animals were treated with CsA, 16 mg/kg/day, beginning the day of surgery. The dose was tapered to 2 mg/kg over 4 weeks, then and maintained at this level. The facial-scalp flaps survived for over 180 days.

With these modifications, a bipedicled composite facial-scalp flap was vascularized by a single common carotid artery of the recipient, without dissecting the other common carotid artery. This modification decreased mortality tremendously by reducing cerebral ischemia time, bleeding, anesthesia time, and complications associated with bilateral common carotid artery dissection, such as vagus and phrenic nerve injuries in the recipients. We believe this pattern of arterial anastomosis would be a good choice in future facial allograft transplants in humans.

Composite Hemifacial Transplant Model

We introduced a hemifacial allograft transplant model, which is less technically challenging then the full-facial allograft transplant. In this model, we investigated the development of operational tolerance across major histocompatibility barriers.

Experimental Model. Composite hemifacial allografts were transplanted from semiallogeneic Lewis- Brown Norway (LBN RT1) and fully allogeneic ACI (RT1[a]) rats to Lewis (RT1) recipients.[51] Composite hemifacial flaps, including the external ear and the scalp, based on the common carotid artery and external jugular vein, were harvested from the left side of the donors. In the recipient, the facial skin on the left side, including external ear, was excised. After setting the flap, the donor external jugular vein was anastomosed end-to-side to the recipient external jugular vein, then the donor carotid artery was anastomosed end-to-side to the recipient common carotid artery.

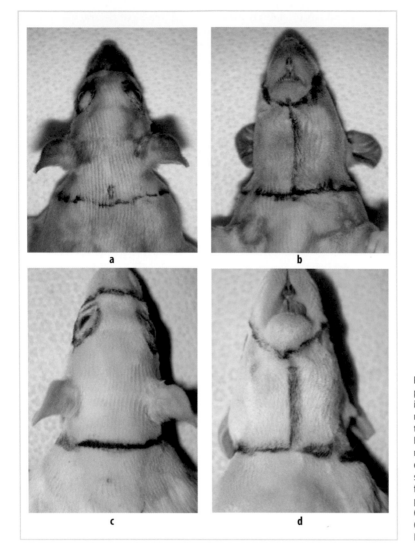

Figure 10-1. The full-facial allograft transplantation model across a major histocompatibility barrier. Preoperative views of the donor rat showing markings of the facial skin flap, the dorsal surface **a** and the ventral surface **b**. Preoperative views of the recipient rat showing markings of the skin to be excised before the donor facial skin transplant inset, the dorsal surface **c** and the ventral surface **d**. (Reprinted from Siemionow MZ, Agaoglu G. Allotransplantation of the Face: How Close Are We? Clinics in Plastic Surgery, Volume 32 (in press). Copyright 2005, with permission from Elsevier.)

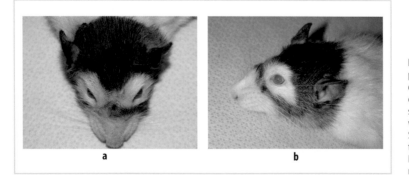

Figure 10-2. The full-facial allograft transplantation model. Late post-transplant views of face allograft recipient on low-dose of cyclosporine A monotherapy at day 200 showing no signs of rejection. **a**) The frontal view. **b**) The lateral view. (Reprinted from Siemionow MZ, Agaoglus G. Allotransplantation of the Face: How Close Are We? Clinics in Plastic Surgery, Volume 32 (in press). Copyright 2005, with permission from Elsevier.)

Immunosuppressive Protocol. Both semialloge-neic and fully allogeneic allograft recipients were treated with standard immunosuppressive protocol of CsA monotherapy, 16 mg/kg/day, which was tapered to 2 mg/kg/day over 4 weeks and maintained at this level thereafter. In this experimental composite hemifacial transplant model, we established operational tolerance and achieved survival rates of 400 days in the semiallogeneic and 330 days in the fully allogeneic MHC mismatched facial transplant recipients (Figure 10-3).

We are encouraged by our success with maintaining total facial-scalp allograft transplants for more than 200 days and by the promising results we achieved in the hemifacial transplant model

using a single immunosuppressive agent therapy without need for recipient conditioning. This experimental knowledge should support future clinical decisions in this challenging procedure.

A Cadaveric Dissection in Preparation for a Human Facial Allograft Transplant

We have dissected cadavers to confirm the feasibility of facial flap harvest and to support the application of facial allograft transplants as a new treatment for patients with severe facial deformities.[55] We compared the potential area of coverage, texture, and color match of these reconstructive options. In 5 cadavers, the com-

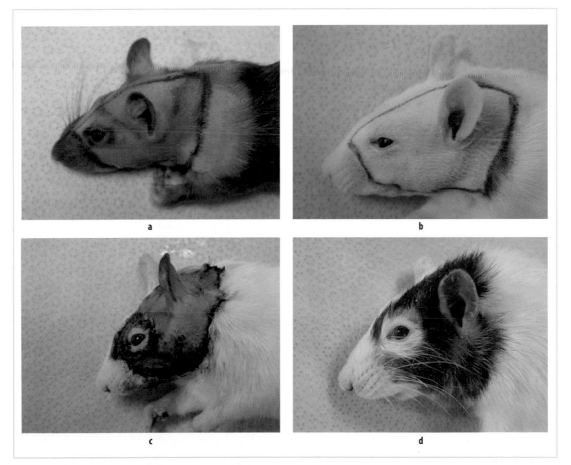

Figure 10-3. The hemi-facial allograft transplantation model. Preoperative view of the donor Lewis-Brown Norway rat showing markings of the facial skin flap **a**). Preoperative view of the recipient Lewis rat showing marking of the skin to be excised before the skin flap inset from the donor **b**). Immedi-ate post-transplant view of the hemiface allograft recipient **c**). The recipient of hemifacial allograft 200 days after transplant shows no signs of rejection on a low maintenance dose of cyclosporine A monotherapy **d**).

posite full-facial–scalp flap was designed to incorporate the entire facial skin, including the skin over the nose, eyelids, lips, both external ears, and the scalp. The flap was elevated in the subplatysmal plane in the neck, in the subsuperficial musculoaponeurotic system plane in the face, and in the subgaleal plane in the scalp. The whole flap was based bilaterally on the external carotid arteries as the arterial pedicles and on the external jugular and facial veins as the venous pedicles (Figures 10-4 and 10-5).

The conventional radial forearm, anterolateral thigh, bipedicled deep inferior epigastric, and bipedicled scapular-parascapular flaps were also harvested from the same cadavers. The total surface areas of the created facial defects and alternative harvested conventional flaps were measured. Methylene blue dye was injected from the external carotid artery for visualization of the facial-scalp vascular network.

The mean surface area for the combined facial-scalp flaps and facial flaps without scalp was $1192\,cm^2$ and $675\,cm^2$, respectively. When compared to the total surface area of the facial-scalp flap, the radial forearm flap covered 13% of the defect, the anterolateral thigh flap 19%, the bipedicled deep inferior epigastric perforator flap 35%, and the bipedicled scapular-parascapular flap 48%, respectively. Coverage of the facial defect without scalp was 24% for the radial forearm flap, 34% for the anterolateral thigh flap, 62% for the bipedicled deep inferior epigastric perforator flap, and 84% for the bipedicled scapular-parascapular flap, respectively (Figure 10-6). The perfused dye was well visualized from the external carotid artery up to the terminal branches of the facial and superficial temporal arteries.

This cadaveric study confirmed that none of the conventional cutaneous autogenous flaps would cover a total facial defect. However, a perfect match of the texture, pliability, and color of facial skin will likely only be achieved by transplanting the facial skin from a human donor.

Mock Facial Transplantation in Preparation for a Human Facial Allograft Transplant

Recently, we have performed a mock facial transplantation by harvesting a total facial-scalp flap from the donor and transferring the flap to the recipient cadavers.[56]

In the donor, we have measured the time of facial-scalp flap harvesting, the length of the arterial and venous pedicles and sensory nerves, which were included in the facial flaps. In the recipient, we have evaluated the time of facial skin harvest as a "monoblock" full-thickness graft, the anchoring regions for the inset of the donor facial flaps and the time sequences for the vascular pedicles anastomoses and nerves coaptations.

In the donor cadaver the mean harvesting time of the total facial-scalp flap harvest was 235.62 ± 21.94 minutes. The mean length of the supraorbital, infraorbital, mental, and great auricular nerves was 1.5 ± 0.15, 2.46 ± 0.25, 3.02 ± 0.31, and $6.11 \pm 0.42\,cm$, respectively. The mean length of the external carotid artery, facial and external jugular veins was 5 ± 0.32, 3.15 ± 0.32, and $5.78 \pm 0.5\,cm$, respectively. In the recipient cadaver the mean harvesting time of facial skin as a "monoblock" full-thickness graft was 47.5 ± 3.53 minutes. The mean time for the preparation of the arterial and venous pedicles and sensory nerves for the future anastomoses and coaptation was 30 ± 0 minutes. The mean time for the facial flap anchoring was 22.5 ± 3.53 minutes. The total mean time of facial mock transplantation without vessels and nerves repair was 320 ± 7.07 minutes (5 hours and 20 minutes).

Based on anatomical dissections in this cadaver study, we have estimated the time and sequence of the facial flap harvest and inset to mimic the clinical scenario of facial transplantation procedure.

Immunosuppressive Strategies in Composite Tissue Allograft Transplants

The development of immunosuppressive agents can be divided into periods before and after the introduction of cyclosporine. Before the CsA era, immunosuppressive regimens were nonselective, consisting mainly of total body or total lymphoid radiation followed by the introduction of 6-mercaptopurine, cyclophosphamide, and azathioprine. Steroids were added to azathioprine to improve effectiveness and reduce toxicity. This combination of steroids and azathioprine, with or without antilymphocyte globulin, was used

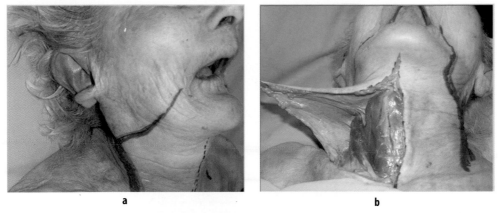

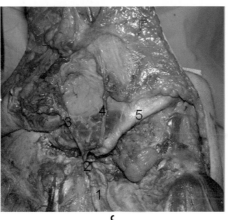

Figure 10-4. Dissection of the facial-scalp flap. **a**) After marking the vascular structure of the flap. **b**) Through a midline incision, the flap was elevated in the subplatysmal plane, including external jugular vein in the flap. (Siemionow MZ, Unal S, Agaoglu G, et al. What are alternative sources for total facial defect coverage? A cadaver study in preparation for facial allograft transplantation in humans. Plastic and Reconstructive Surgery (PRS-D-04-00324, in press) 2005.)

c) Elevation of the flap showing arterial network of the flap. 1) The common carotid artery. 2) The external carotid artery. 3) The superficial temporal artery. 4) The facial artery. 5) The lower border of mandible. (Reprinted from Siemionow MZ, Agaoglu G. Allotransplantation of the Face: How Close Are We? Clinics in Plastic Surgery, Volume 32 (in press). Copyright 2005, with permission from Elsevier.)

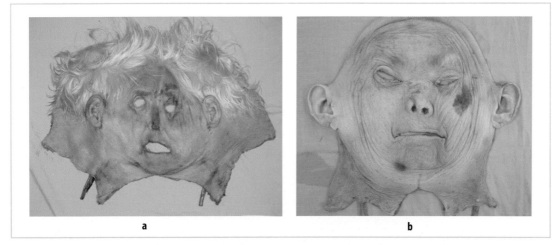

Figure 10-5. a) Harvested total facial-scalp flap. **b**) Harvested facial flap without scalp. (Siemionow MZ, Unal S, Agaoglu G, et al. What are alternative sources for total facial defect coverage? A cadaver study in preparation for facial allograft transplantation in humans. Plastic and Reconstructive Surgery (PRS-D-04-00324, in press) 2005.)

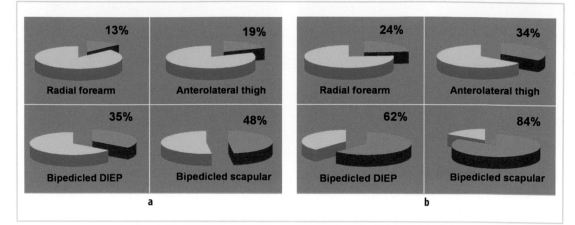

Figure 10-6. Outline of the percentage of the conventional flaps that covers the surface area of **a**) a total facial scalp defect and **b**) a facial defect without scalp.

for about 2 decades, until a new era of immuno-suppression was begun with the introduction of CsA. Cyclosporine was the first specific drug to target T cells by inhibiting T-cell-mediated IL-2 production, a crucial cytokine for T-cell expansion. Thereafter, several new agents targeted T cells, interleukin receptors, and various T-cell receptors, such as monoclonal antibodies (OKT3), calcineurin inhibitors (FK506), nucleic acid inhibitors (mycophenolate mofetil (MMF)) and inhibitors of signals for T-cell differentiation (sirolimus).[48,57,58]

Composite tissue allografts, unlike solid organs, contain different types of tissue with variable degrees of antigenicity. Thus, to be successful, any immunosuppressive protocol should prevent rejection of all these tissues.

Different immunosuppressive protocols were used in both experimental and clinical CTA transplantations.

Experimental Immunosuppressive Protocols

Experiments on animals show that donor-specific tolerance can be achieved through stable mixed allogeneic chimerism after bone marrow transplantation. Most of the experimental studies on CTA transplants have been performed on rodents. Different immunosuppressive agents have been used as a monotherapy or in combination protocols. In our laboratory, in a rat hind limb transplantation model, with only a short-term therapy of combined CsA and $\alpha\beta$-T-cell receptor monoclonal antibody, we were able to induce long-term, donor-specific tolerance across a MHC barrier, obtaining long-term survival of the animals over 350 days without recipient conditioning and the need for chronic immunosuppression. Tolerance was confirmed by skin grafting in vivo and mixed lymphocyte reaction in vitro. The animals rejected third-party grafts, which indicate immunocompetence.[47]

Limited numbers of experiments have been done on large animals to evaluate the efficacy of various immunosuppressive protocols on CTA transplants. In a swine model of limb transplantation, the antirejection effects of different immunosuppressive protocols were assessed including CsA alone, CsA/MMF, and FK506-MMF.[59-61] The FK506-MMF combination was the most successful in preventing allograft rejection and was considered to be a clinically applicable treatment,[59] but it was associated with more toxicity when compared to CsA/MMF protocol therapy.[60]

Primates are the most reliable models for CTA transplantation because they are closely related to humans. Primates have been used only in few studies as a model of CTA transplants, and the most commonly used immunosuppressive agents were CsA and steroids.[62,63]

Clinical Immunosuppressive Protocols

Lifelong immunosuppression is one of the important issues that need to be discussed with patients considering facial transplantation. Standard transplantation protocols include nonspecific immunosuppressive drugs. The number of these drugs is increasing every year, and this large number may offer an opportunity to find ideal regimens.

Immunosuppressive protocols consist of induction and maintenance therapies to prevent allograft rejection and short courses of intensive therapies to suppress acute episodes of rejection. Currently, the immunosuppressive drugs used in the induction protocols of immunosuppression for CTA transplantation mainly include steroids, antithymocyte globulin (ATG), and OKT3, whereas maintenance protocols of immunosuppression include, calcineurin inhibitors (CsA and FK506), mycophenolate mofetil (MMF), and steroids.

Solid organ transplantation is essential for life; therefore, both patient and society usually accept the side effects of immunosuppressive agents. However, facial allograft transplantation is intended to improve the quality of life, rather than to save it. It is hard to quantify the benefits of facial allograft transplantation or the risk of lifelong immunosuppression, so decisions about this procedure should be made on individual basis and should be based on the type of composite tissue to be transplanted.

The patient has to be informed about the side effects of immunosuppressive protocols, as well as of the need to adhere to these protocols for life. The first hand transplant was re-amputated because of the patient's nonadherence with physical therapy and immunosuppressive treatment.[27] This case shows the importance of patient selection and adherence to immunosuppressive therapy.

Although great advances have been made in immunosuppressive therapies, immunosuppressive agents are still associated with significant side effects including: organ toxicity, lifethreatening viral and fungal infections, and malignancies.[64,65] Commonly used calcineurin inhibitors in induction and maintenance therapy have similar side effects on renal and hepatic function. Neurotoxic effects and post-transplant diabetes mellitus are higher under tacrolimus protocols, whereas the risks of hypercholesterolemia and hypertension are lower compared to those with CsA. Tacrolimus promotes nerve regeneration,[66] so this agent will be preferred in CTA transplantations because nerve regeneration will be one of the goals after transplantation.

Steroids are commonly used, both in induction and maintenance protocols of immunosuppression for CTA. Tapering the dose to the lower maintenance dosage, especially when initially given in higher dosages, can reduce systemic toxic effects. However, the main issue in implementing steroid protocols for CTA transplants is the need for higher induction dosages, which will have negative effects on the wound healing. Therefore, low prednisone dosage in the early postoperative period will be critical for CTA transplant protocols.

Immunosuppression-related complications can be prevented by close monitoring of the patients and by early medical intervention. The immunologic side effects can be managed by switching the type of immunosuppressant, which was the case after larynx transplantation, where CsA was exchanged with tacrolimus to control hypertension associated with nephrotoxicity.[33]

The side effects of immunosuppression have raised concern about the risk-benefit ratio of CTA transplantations that are not life-saving. However, transplantation of a facial allograft is distinct from other CTA transplants. The sociopsychological benefits of face transplantation may offset the potential risks of lifelong immunosuppression.

When lifelong immunosuppressive therapy will not be necessary, and tolerance-inducing strategies would be available, transplantation of the face would be considered for patients with severe facial deformities. In the near future, standard tolerance inducing protocols will likely be introduced, opening a new era for facial and other CTA transplants.

Psychological, Social, and Ethical Considerations of Facial Transplantation

Advances in the field of reconstructive surgery and recent success in CTA transplantation have made facial allograft transplantation for patients with severe facial deformities the next step in the field of CTA transplantation. Since the first announcement to consider facial transplantation, excited discussions regarding the ethical, social and psychological issues began in the medical community. The number of candidates who would benefit from facial allograft transplantation is limited. Candidates should be evaluated by a multidisciplinary team that should include plastic surgeons, transplant surgeons, immunologists, psychiatrists, psychologists, infectious disease specialists, ethicists, patient advocates, social workers, lawyers for the medical community, and public relations experts.

Facial transplantation should be considered as a medical solution to relieve the suffering of severely disfigured patients. The psychological and social consequences of this procedure can be foreseen, but unfortunately, the final outcome cannot be predicted.[67,68] In general, organ transplantation may lead to a group of stresses and psychosocial problems. Fears and anxiety related to organ viability, the possibility of the graft rejection, and the probability of toxic effects of immunosuppressive agents is well documented after organ transplantation. Feelings of gratefulness and guilt concerning the donor's family are among other emotional responses in patients with organ transplants.[69] These fears and anxieties would likely be amplified in the case of facial transplantation by factors such as issues of identity and communication, psychological vulnerability and resilience, motivation to seek treatment, expectations of outcome, consequences of transplant failure, adherence to treatment regimens, and dealing with the reactions of others to altered appearance.[41] The defect created in the donor after facial flap harvesting may be not acceptable to the donor or the donor's family. Consequently, finding of a facial transplant donor will probably be very difficult, compared to achieving consent for solid organ donation. Thus, specific "reconstructive" options should also be considered for the donor and should be discussed with the family. Options for the coverage of created defects would include full-thickness skin grafts or synthetic materials, including silicone masks. All these options, as well as the possibility of closed-casket funeral, should be discussed with the donor's family.

The First Institutional Review Board Approval for Facial Transplants

On October 15, 2004, the Cleveland Clinic Foundation's Institutional Review Board approved the first protocol for facial allograft transplantation in humans. Presented by Dr. Maria Siemionow, the protocol required 10 months of debate on the medical, ethical, and psychological issues. The inclusion and exclusion criteria for screening potential candidates for facial transplantation were thoroughly evaluated. The donor and recipient consent forms have been approved. This IRB approval allowed us to open the Facial Transplantation Program, where teams of specialists, including surgeons, psychologists, psychiatrists, ethicists, patient advocates, and media representatives will evaluate patients with severe facial deformities. Based on this evaluation, the most appropriate candidates for facial transplantation will be selected.

The question remains whether potential donors and the donor's families will ever accept facial skin donation. At this point, we are not sure how close we are or how long it will take for the first facial transplantation to be done. It may not happen for 6 months or a year. It may not happen in our lifetime. But it may also happen sooner than we expect.

Conclusion

Patients living with severe facial deformities may wish to assume the risks of allograft transplantation if they have the chance to obtain a more normal appearance. Facial allograft transplantation would revolutionize the field of transplantation and reconstructive surgery. The advantages and disadvantages of this promising procedure should thoroughly be discussed with recipients and their families (Table 10-1). Although the likelihood of success

Table 10-1. Advantages and Disadvantages of Facial Allograft Transplantation

Advantages	Disadvantages
• No donor site morbidity • Complete facial reconstruction in single surgical procedure • Option for total external ear replacement or reconstruction • Better skin texture, pliability, and color match	• Adequate matching between the donor and recipient is difficult (age, sex, race) • Lifelong immunosuppression • Increased risks of comorbidities (diabetes, infections, lymphoproliferative disorder, avascular necrosis of bones) • Social, ethical, and psychological issues

and the long-term functional and esthetic results remain unclear at this time, facial allograft transplantation will someday become a reality. When this time comes, we believe that well informed and psychologically stable patients should have right to decide whether to undergo this procedure.

References

1. Ergun SS, Cek DI, Demirkesen C. Is facial resurfacing with monobloc full-thickness skin graft a remedy in xeroderma pigmentosum? *Plast Reconstr Surg.* 2002; 110:1290–1293.

2. Ashall G, Quaba AA, Hackett ME. Facial resurfacing in xeroderma pigmentosum: are we spoiling the ship for a ha'p'orth of tar? *Br J Plast Surg.* 1987;40:610–613.

3. Erol OO. The transformation of a free skin graft into a vascularized pedicle flap. *Plast Reconstr Surg.* 1976;58: 470–477.

4. Pribaz JJ, Fine N, Orgill DP. Flap prefabrication in the head and neck: a 10-year experience. *Plast Reconstr Surg.* 1999;103:808–820.

5. Khouri RK, Upton J, Shaw WW. Prefabrication of composite free flaps through staged microvascular transfer: an experimental and clinical study. *Plast Reconstr Surg.* 1991;87:108–115.

6. Teot L, Cherenfant E, Otman S, et al. Prefabricated vascularised supraclavicular flaps for face resurfacing after postburns scarring. *Lancet.* 2000;355:1695–1696.

7. Boyd JB. Tissue expansion in reconstruction. *South Med J.* 1987;80:430–432.

8. Wilmshurst AD, Sharpe DT. Immediate placement of tissue expanders in the management of large excisional defects on the face. *Br J Plast Surg.* 1990;43:150–153.

9. Kawashima T, Yamada A, Ueda K, et al. Tissue expansion in facial reconstruction. *Plast Reconstr Surg.* 1994; 94:944–950.

10. Spence RJ. Experience with novel uses of tissue expanders in burn reconstruction of the face and neck. *Ann Plast Surg.* 1992;28:453–464.

11. Harii K, Ohmori K, Ohmori S. Utilization of free composite tissue transfer by microvascular anastomosis for the repair of burn deformities. *Burn.* 1975;1:237–244.

12. Burget GC, Menick FJ. The subunit principle in nasal reconstruction. *Plast Reconstr Surg.* 1985;76:239–247.

13. Feldman JJ. Facial resurfacing: the single sheet concept. In: Brent B, editor. *The Artistry of Plastic Surgery.* St. Louis: Mosby, 1987.

14. Angrigiani C, Grilli D. Total face reconstruction with one free flap. *Plast Reconstr Surg.* 1997;99:1566–1575.

15. Miller GD, Auster EJ, Shell JA. Successful replantation of an avulsed scalp by microsurgical anastomoses. *Plast Reconstr Surg.* 1976;58:133–136.

16. Cheng K, Zhou S, Jiang K, et al. Replantation of the avulsed scalp: report of 20 cases. *Plast Reconstr Surg.* 1996;97:1099–1106.

17. Hammond DC, Bouwense C, Hankins WT, et al. Microsurgical replantation of the amputated nose. *Plast Reconstr Surg.* 2000;105:2133–2136.

18. Concannon MJ, Puckett CL. Microsurgical replantation of an ear in a child without venous repair. *Plast Reconstr Surg.* 1998;102:2088–2093.

19. Jeng SF, Wei FC, Noordhoff MS. Successful replantation of a bitten-off vermilion of the lower lip by microvascular anastomosis: case report. *J Trauma.* 1992;33:914–916.

20. Thomas A, Obed V, Murarka A, et al. Total face and scalp replantation. *Plast Reconstr Surg.* 1998;102:2085–2087.

21. Wilhelmi BJ, Kang RH, Movassaghi K, et al. First successful replantation of face and scalp with single-artery repair: model for face and scalp transplantation. *Ann Plast Surg.* 2003;50:535–540.

22. Kahan BD. Cosmas and Damian in the 20th century? *N Engl J Med.* 1981;305:280–281.

23. Dubernard JM, Owen E, Herzberg G, et al. Human hand allograft: report on first 6 months. *Lancet.* 1999;353:1315–1320.

24. Petit F, Minns AB, Dubernard JM, et al. Composite tissue allotransplantation and reconstructive surgery: first clinical applications. *Ann Surg.* 2003;237: 19–25.

25. Cendales L, Breidenbach W, Granger DK, et al. Evaluation of function following human hand transplantation [Abstract]. *Transplantation.* 2000;69:S295.

26. Jones JW, Gruber SA, Barker JH, et al. Successful hand transplantation. One-year follow-up. *N Engl J Med.* 2000;343:468–473.

27. Francois CG, Breidenbach WC, Maldonado C, et al. Hand transplantation: comparisons and observations of the first four clinical cases. *Microsurgery.* 2000;20:360–371.

28. Hettiaratchy S, Randolph MA, Petit F, et al. Composite tissue allotransplantation—a new era in plastic surgery? *Br J Plast Surg.* 2004;57:381–391.

29. Levi DM, Tzakis AG, Kato T, et al. Transplantation of the abdominal wall. *Lancet.* 2003;36:2173–2176.

30. Hofmann GO, Kirschner MH, Wagner FD, et al. Allogeneic vascularized transplantation of human femoral diaphyses and total knee joints—first clinical experiences. *Transplant Proc.* 1998;30:2754–2761.

31. Mackinnon SE, Doolabh VB, Novak CB, et al. Clinical outcome following nerve allograft transplantation. *Plast Reconstr Surg.* 2001; 107:1419–1429.

32. Guimberteau JC, Baudet J, Panconi B, et al. Human allo-transplant of a digital flexion system vascularized on the ulnar pedicle: a preliminary report and 1-year follow up of two cases. *Plast Reconstr Surg.* 1992; 89: 1135–1147.

33. Strome M, Stein J, Esclamado R, et al. Laryngeal transplantation and 40-month follow-up. *N Engl J Med.* 2001;344:1676–1679.

34. Jones TR, Humphrey PA, Brennan DC. Transplantation of vascularized allogeneic skeletal muscle for scalp reconstruction in a renal transplant patient. *Transplant Proc.* 1998;30:2746–2753.

35. Birchall M. Tongue transplantation. *Lancet.* 2004;363: 1663.

36. Denton MD, Magee CC, Sayegh MH. Immunosuppressive strategies in transplantation. *Lancet.* 1999;353: 1083–1091.

37. Elster EA, Xu H, Tadaki DK, et al. Treatment with the humanized CD154-specific monoclonal antibody, hu5C8, prevents acute rejection of primary skin allografts in nonhuman primates. *Transplantation.* 2001;72:1473–1478.

38. Knechtle SJ. Treatment with immunotoxin. *Philos Trans R Soc Lond B Biol Sci.* 2001;356:681–689.

39. Spitzer TR, Delmonico F, Tolkoff-Rubin N, et al. Combined histocompatibility leukocyte antigen-matched donor bone marrow and renal transplantation for multiple myeloma with end stage renal disease: the induction of allograft tolerance through mixed lymphohematopoietic chimerism. *Transplantation.* 1999; 68:480–484.

40. Buncke HJ, Hoffman WY, Alpert BS, et al. Microvascular transplant of two free scalp flaps between identical twins. *Plast Reconstr Surg.* 1982;70:605–609.

41. Morris PJ, Bradley JA, Doyal L, et al. Facial transplantation: a working party report from the Royal College of Surgeons of England. *Transplantation.* 2004;77:330–338.

42. Ozer K, Izycki D, Zielinski M, et al. Development of donor-specific chimerism and tolerance in composite tissue allografts under alphabeta-T-cell receptor monoclonal antibody and cyclosporine a treatment protocols. *Microsurgery.* 2004;24:248–254.

43. Siemionow M, Izycki DM, Zielinski M. Donor-specific tolerance in fully major histocompatibility major histocompatibility complex-mismatched limb allograft transplants under an anti-alphabeta T-cell receptor monoclonal antibody and cyclosporine A protocol. *Transplantation.* 2003;76:1662–1668.

44. Ozer K, Gurunluoglu R, Zielinski M, et al. Extension of composite tissue allograft survival across major histocompatibility barrier under short course of anti-lymphocyte serum and cyclosporine a therapy. *J Reconstr Microsurg.* 2003;19:249–56.

45. Ozer K, Oke R, Gurunluoglu R, et al. Induction of tolerance to hind limb allografts in rats receiving cyclosporine A and antilymphocyte serum: effect of duration of the treatment. *Transplantation.* 2003;75:31–36.

46. Siemionow M, Oke R, Ozer K, et al. Induction of donor-specific tolerance in rat hind-limb allografts under anti-lymphocyte serum and cyclosporine A protocol. *J Hand Surg* [Am]. 2002;27:1095–1103.

47. Siemionow M, Ortak T, Izycki D, et al. Induction of tolerance in composite-tissue allografts. *Transplantation.* 2002;15:1211–1217.

48. Siemionow M, Ozer K. Advances in composite tissue allograft transplantation as related to the hand and upper extremity. *J Hand Surg* [Am]. 2002;27:565–568.

49. Siemionow M, Gozel-Ulusal B, Ulusal A, et al. Functional tolerance following face transplantation in the rat. *Transplantation.* 2003;75:1607–1609.

50. Ulusal BG, Ulusal AE, Ozmen S, et al. A new composite facial and scalp transplantation model in rats. *Plast Reconstr Surg.* 2003;112:1302–1311.

51. Demir Y, Ozmen S, Klimczak A, et al. Tolerance induction in composite facial allograft transplantation in the rat model. *Plast Reconstr Surg.* 2004;114:1790–1801.

52. Demir Y, Ozmen S, Klimczak A, et al. The efficacy of different immunosuppressive treatment protocols on survival and development of chimerism in vascularized skin allograft transplants across MHC barrier. *Plast Reconstr Surg.* (In press).

53. Unal S, Agaoglu G, Siemionow M. New surgical approach in facial transplantation extends survival of allograft recipients. *Ann Plast Surg.* In press.

54. Bermudez LE, Santamaria A, Romero T, et al. Experimental model of facial transplant. *Plast Reconstr Surg.* 2002;110:1374–1375.

55. Siemionow M, Unal S, Agaoglu G, et al. What are alternative sources for total facial defect coverage? A cadaver study in preparation for facial allograft transplantation in humans–part I. *Plast Reconstr Surg.* In press.

56. Siemionow S, Agaoglu G, Unal S. Mock facial transplantation a cadaver study in preparation for facial allograft transplantation in humans, part II. *Plast Reconstr Surg.* In press.

57. Gorantla VS, Barker JH, Jones JW Jr, et al. Immunosuppressive agents in transplantation: mechanisms of action and current anti-rejection strategies. *Microsurgery.* 2000;20:420–429.

58. Cendales L, Hardy MA. Immunologic considerations in composite tissue transplantation: overview. *Microsurgery.* 2000;20:412–419.

59. Jones JW Jr, Ustuner ET, Zdichavsky M, et al. Long-term survival of an extremity composite tissue allograft with FK506-mycophenolate mofetil therapy. *Surgery.* 1999; 126:384–388.

60. Ustuner ET, Zdichavsky M, Ren X, et al. Long-term composite tissue allograft survival in a porcine model with cyclosporine/mycophenolate mofetil therapy. *Transplantation.* 1998;66:1581–1587.

61. Lee WP, Rubin JP, Cober S, et al. Use of swine model in transplantation of vascularized skeletal tissue allografts. *Transplant Proc.* 1998;30:2743–2745.

62. Stark GB, Swartz WM, Narayanan K, et al. Hand transplantation in baboons. *Transplant Proc.* 1987;19:3968–3971.

63. Hovius SE, Stevens HP, van Nierop PW, et al. Allogeneic transplantation of the radial side of the hand in the rhesus monkey: I. technical aspects. *Plast Reconstr Surg.* 1992;89:700–709.

64. Miller LW. Cardiovascular toxicities of immunosuppressive agents. *Am J Transplantation.* 2002;2:807–818.

65. Euvrard S, Kanitakis J, Claudy A. Skin cancer after organ transplantation. *N Engl J Med.* 2003;343:1681–1691.

66. Jost SC, Doolabh VB, Mackinnon SE, et al. Accelera-tion of peripheral nerve regeneration following FK506 administration. *Restor Neurol Neurosci.* 2000;17:39–44.

67. Siemionow M, Ozmen S, Demir Y. Prospects for facial allograft transplantation in humans. *Plast Reconstr Surg.* 2004;113:1421–1428.

68. Petit F, Paraskevas A, Minns AB, et al. Face transplantation: where do we stand? *Plast Reconstr Surg.* 2004; 113:1429–1433.

69. Ziegelmann J, Griva K, Hankins M, et al. The transplant effects questionnaire; the development of a questionnaire for assessing the multidimensional outcome of organ transplantation—example of end stage renal disease (ESRD). *Br J Health Psychol.* 2000;7: 393–408.

11

Tissue Engineering: Current Approaches and Future Directions

Amir H. Ajar and Gregory R.D. Evans

Introduction

Tissue engineering marries the fields of engineering and life sciences with the goal of fashioning biomimetic materials to augment, restore, or maintain biologic systems after damage by disease or injury. That is, tissue engineering seeks replicate the functions usually performed by the body's organs; a goal sometimes referred to as "the missing organ problem."[1]

Six basic methods of tissue engineering have been described: 1) transplantation, 2) autografting, 3) prosthesis, 4) stem cell generation, 5) in-vitro tissue engineering, and 6) in-vivo tissue engineering. These methods have been further stratified into substitutive, histioconductive, and histioinductive approaches, which are based on either developing ex-vivo materials (substitutive and histioconductive) or on facilitating self-repair of damaged tissue (histioinductive).[2]

To achieve effective, long-lasting repair of damaged tissues, any of the above methods of tissue engineering must meet at least 5 criteria: 1) the number of cells or the size of tissue generated must be sufficient to accomplish the repair, 2) cells must be appropriately differentiated toward the desired phenotype, 3) the extracellular matrix must maintain an appropriate three-dimensional organization and be adequately supported, 4) cells and tissues must be structurally and mechanically compliant with the normal demands of native tissue, and 5) cells and tissues must be fully integrated with native tissue.[3]

Any consideration of tissue engineering should, however, be made in the context of current therapies for treating tissue injury, as well their inherent limitations. Presently, synthetic biomaterials, autografting, and allografting have numerous applications, from joint and vessel replacement to skin grafting and organ transplantation. However, synthetic biomaterials, such as Dacron, polytetrafluoroethylene (PTFE), titanium alloy, and ceramics elicit foreign-body reactions and are limited in the long-term by their inability to grow and remodel in the recipient host. Autografting, by definition, suffers from a potential paucity of adequate quality or quantity of graftable tissue, as well as by donor-site morbidity. Allografting, regardless of continuing efforts at tightening safeguards, carries the ever-present risk of disease transmission and immune rejection.

The challenge of tissue engineering therefore becomes how to create a stable, infection-free, biocompatible material that displays the dynamic, in-vivo properties of the tissue it intends to replace, either alone or in conjunction with modulation of biologic systems, to maximize native tissue repair. In this chapter, we review 3 tissue engineering techniques being developed toward this end: stem cells, polymers, and growth factors.

Stem Cells

Using stem cells in tissue engineering makes intuitive sense and has great promise. Stem cells are, by definition, multipotent and self-regenerating, giving them the unique potential of maintaining cellular homeostasis in functional tissue for the lifetime of the organism.

To be applicable for tissue engineering, the stem cell must first be differentiated into the lineage-committed cell type of the tissue of interest. They must then assemble into an appropriate three-dimensional architecture dictated by the functional requirements of the tissue in question. To understand the potential of stem cells toward this end, several principles of stem cell physiology merit discussion.

Stem cells can be divided into two main classes, the first of which is the pluripotent stem cells, which are capable of assuming all types of tissue, except extra-embryonic membranes, making them incapable of generating embryonic tissue. Pluripotent cells are found as embryonic stem cells in the inner cell mass of the blastocyst, as well as in germ cells of the gonadal ridge in the fetus.[4,5] Embryonic stem and germ cells differ in several ways, including the conditions required for isolation, population doublings, and survivability in cell culture, with embryonic stem cells being overall the more robust of the two.[6] Embryonic stem cells can be manipulated into a wide-range of cell types, including muscle cells, neural cells, vascular endothelium, and endodermal derivatives.[7] Although the molecular mechanisms of in-vitro self-renewal have been described in murine cell populations, the mechanisms of human embryonic stem cell regulation remain unknown.[8]

The second major class of stem cell is the multipotent stem cell, which is considered to be the offspring of pluripotent cells and to be directed into more specific cell lineages. In other words, multipotent stem cells are less plastic and more differentiated than their pluripotent counterparts. A common source of multipotent stem cells is the adult human, and the most extensively characterized are the bone marrow-derived stem cells. These cells consist of two distinct stem cell populations: 1) hematopoietic stem cells, which are responsible for the development of the entire blood cell line, including white blood cells, red blood cells, and platelets; and 2) mesenchymal stem cells, which give rise to numerous connective tissues, including bone, cartilage, adipose, muscle, tendon, and neural tissue in both in-vitro and in-vivo settings.[9] Mesenchymal stem cells are present in adult bone marrow, fat, muscle, and skin.[10]

Applications of Stem Cells in Tissue Repair

A recent review of stem cell research for tissue repair reported encouraging results from early experiments using embryonic stem cells from rats and mice to repair nerve and muscle tissue.

Efforts to seed human embryonic stem cell derivatives into human beings are ongoing.[11] Adding to the challenge of human clinical use is recent evidence that MHC class 1 proteins, found on the surface of all nucleated cells responsible for antigen presentation to T cells, are expressed on human embryonic stem cells which increase after differentiation. This makes tissue rejection by the host all the more likely.[12] Ways to minimize this untoward effect include developing an "embryonic stem cell bank" that could match cells to individual patients; genetically altering cells to develop a "universal donor" that does not express MHC proteins, and developing nuclear transfer techniques to derive genetically matched stem cells for individual patients.[13]

Adult stem cells, as mentioned earlier, have the ability to differentiate into numerous cell lineages. The assumption that their function would be limited to those of the cell lineages present in the organ of original harvest has not held true. To date, adult bone marrow, brain, skeletal muscle, liver, pancreas, fat, and skin all have been shown to possess progenitor cells capable of differentiating into cell types other than their tissue of native origin.[11] Stem cells introduced into a novel environment are now believed to undergo "reprogramming" in response to local signals elaborated by their new surroundings, although this reprogramming is poorly understood.[12]

A better understanding of these cellular mechanisms has come from studies of synthetic microenvironments that clarify the role of matrix, growth factor, and cellular adhesion cues in stem cell differentiation and histogenesis.[14] In these studies, local levels of both soluble and insoluble molecules were sustained at the site of cell transplantation. In this particular case, the brain was the tissue model in question. Transplantable "neo-tissues" were created using cells assembled with cell-adhesive and controlled-release microparticles, with growth factor dosing and subsequent effect being controlled by varying either the number of distributed microparticles or the rate at which growth factor was released from these microparticles.[14] As such, these "neo-tissues" were effectively shown to be "programmable." Assessing cell viability has been the source of extensive research, with local cell viability being determined with the model of three-dimensional, engineered skeletal muscle constructs. Using dual fluorescent staining and confocal laser scanning microscopy, the viability of these constructs was determined after calibrating the average fluoroscopic intensity per living cell.[15] While likely to be limited by the thickness of the engineered tissue and amount of cellular proliferation present in the sample, this technique represents a potential advance in nondestructive quantitative analysis of in-vitro tissue constructs.[15]

Biomaterials

Recent interest in biodegradable polymers and other materials has led to an exciting expansion of potential treatments, either alone or in conjunction with other methods of tissue engineering. Biodegradable products are thought to have at least two potential advantages. First, a substance able to be effectively cleared by the body would not have to be removed after use by secondary surgery. Second, the progressive loss of mechanical strength of the material could conceivably mimic the natural healing process.[16] These advantages, however, come with a large number of other considerations, namely, molecular weight, chemical composition, morphology, additives, and environmental conditions. Success of an engineered tissue construct in turn becomes in large part the product of the interaction of these bio-scaffolds and cells, either in situ or mobilized in vitro. In the segment to follow, natural and synthetic polymers, as well as injectable hydrogels will be discussed in the context of tissue engineering and wound repair.

Early work with chondrocytes revealed the importance of an agarose scaffold in redifferentiating cells during the expansion phase.[17] Since this time, research toward engineering tissue scaffolds for bioengineering applications has followed four general principles: 1) defining a space that will shape the regenerating tissue; 2) adopting a temporary function in a defect while native tissue regenerates; 3) facilitating tissue ingrowth; and 4) including seeded cells, proteins, genes, or all 3 to accelerate wound healing.[18]

Perhaps the largest and most prolific area of research in polymer scaffolds remains in the domain of skeletal tissue engineering. A recent review of the literature by Lu et al. discusses important aspects of scaffold design, materials, and processing of skeletal tissue constructs, which in many circumstances parallel the polymer characteristics used for other applications of tissue engineering.[19]

Beginning with design, a basic requirement of polymeric scaffolds is biocompatibility. Factors affecting this requirement include the chemistry and morphology of the construct, as well as the process of synthesis itself. Residual chemicals from processing have the potential of leaching from the scaffold and adversely affecting both the tissue construct and the native tissue in the vicinity of the implant. The property of biodegradability of the polymer scaffold itself is not, however, sufficient to be clinically applicable when designing polymeric scaffolds. Several cases have been reported in which tissue necrosis or untoward inflammation in the area of implantation has occurred as a direct result of polymer degradation by natural host mechanisms that in turn jeopardize the overall viability of the repair.[19] As a result, precise accounting of the mechanism of polymer biodegradability is an absolute requirement for successful tissue engineering applications.

Polymer engineering aims to construct a scaffold that provides the cellular stability necessary to encourage maximal cellular proliferation with the intention of appropriate extracellular matrix generation. This extracellular matrix in turn replaces the polymeric scaffold originally in place, as it becomes absorbed and excreted by the body. The critical structural variables of the cellular environment necessary to establish and maintain tissue form and function remain to be identified. Toward this end, structure–mechanical analysis of cells and their supporting scaffold within tissue constructs are being investigated in three dimensions using confocal microscopy in reflection mode (backscattered light) to selectively visualize microstructural deformation of the scaffold. The deformation observed at both macro- and microscopic levels during the application of controlled, quantified mechanical loads in turn allows for accurate characterization of structural-mechanical relationships between biomaterials and cell-scaffold constructs.[20] The materials for polymer scaffolds are numerous and depend to a large extent on the indication of the tissue construct in question. Natural polymers, such as starch-based polymers, are effective platforms for murine fibroblast cell growth.[21] Chitosan, a partially deacetylated derivative of chitin, itself a natural polymer product of insects, worms, crustaceans, and fungi, has been proved to be clinically useful as a biomaterial. Chitosan-calcium phosphate polymers are being studied for humanlike osteoblast growth, and chitosan-thioglycolic acid conjugates have shown in-situ gelling properties at physiologic temperatures and pH with specific shapes similar to native tissue.[22,23]

Collagen is the major component of the extracellular matrix; collagen fibers have been described as scaffolding biomaterial for ligamentous replacement, whereas collagen-chondroitin sulfate matrix promotes chondrocyte proliferation and differentiation in vitro.[24,25] Newer, solid free-form fabrication techniques, involving the construction of three-dimensional objects of desired shapes using layered manufacturing strategies, along with critical-point drying (the exchange of ethanol with liquid carbon dioxide at set pressure), can be used to create predefined and reproducible pores of various sizes and interconnections in collagen scaffolds for optimal transport of nutrients and oxygen to the construct.[26]

Synthetic polymers are also commonly used in research, which has produced at least one clinically useful product, Dermagraft (polylactide co-glycolide). However, synthetic polymers are limited by physical properties that adversely affect their degradation profiles, including a tendency to crumble, inciting mechanical damage to tissues, as well as foreign body tissue reactions.[27] As a result, researchers are now taking aim at "semi-synthetic" polymer derivatives, which may address the shortcomings of synthetic constructs while simultaneously improving on and tailoring natural polymers to the application of interest. For example, chitosan-polyglycolide hybrids can maintain fibroblast viability and spindle morphology in culture experiments.[28] The resemblance of chitosan to the components of proteoglycans is conducive to cellular attachment and constitutional function, and polyglycolic acid serves as an effective scaffold with its exceptional biocompatible and biodegradable profile. Similarly, starch blended with ethylene vinyl alcohol (named SEVA-C), when reinforced with synthetic hydroxyapatite, formed a calcium phosphate layer on its surface in situ, giving the construct the potential to bond bone when implanted in vivo.[29]

An alternative to the polymeric scaffolds described above are the more recent tissue engineering approaches employing injectable, in-situ gel-forming matrix systems. Such a delivery system has advantages over more "conventional" polymer scaffold techniques, including the ability to fill a defect of any shape, the incorporation of various therapeutic agents, the lack of residual solvents, and nonsurgical placement.[30] By definition, a gel is a three-dimensional network swollen by a solvent that can be classified according to the fashion of the network to which it is connected; either by chemical (covalent bonds) or physical forces. These gel polymers are capable of incorporating water without dissolving the polymer, giving them the characteristics of soft tissue and a high permeability for oxygen, nutrients, and water-soluble metabolites.[31] Four main classes of injectable gel systems have been investigated to date. They are thermoreversible, pH-reversible, ionically cross-linked, and high-viscosity, shear-thinning gels.

Thermoreversible gels undergo phase transition with increasing temperature when the polymer concentration is above a critical value. A synthetic example is polyethylene oxide-b-propylene oxide-b-ethylene oxide (PEO-PPO-PEO), which has recently been applied to form a cartilage layer on host bone, as well as injected to form cartilage in mice.[32] The pH-reversible gels, such as chitosans, are charged, water-soluble gel-forming polymers in response to pH shifts that have been studied as injectable, resorbable templates in bone regeneration.[30] Ionically cross-linked gels are water-soluble charged polymers that form gels when the react with di- or trivalent ions (e.g., alginate). Although in-vivo experiments have successfully employed alginate to deliver autologous chondrocytes, the risk of enhanced immunogenicity and poor bioresorbability have raised concerns over the possibility of adverse tissue reactions.[30,33] High-viscosity shear-thinning gels, of which hyaluronic acid is representative, can be introduced into tissue through small-bore needles and can subsequently form thick gels once the shear force from the injection has been removed. This property has been manipulated to repair contour deficits in the skin non-operatively.[30] A commercially available hyaluronic acid product, Restylane, has been used to augment the lip but is not yet approved by the FDA. Most recently, synthetic materials have been developed that are capable of assisting tissue regeneration by mimicking matrix metalloproteinase-mediated invasion of native extracellular matrix.[34] In a critical size defect in a calvarial bone model, this synthetic gel underwent a cell-mediated mechanism of matrix breakdown, which occurred in temporal and spatial synchrony with endogenous bone regeneration. In contrast, more conventional biodegradable gel polymers are denatured by chemical pathways, independent of cellular invasion and repair.

An interesting addendum to gel engineering, is a newer approach to generating gel polymers for tissue engineering applications: photopolymerization. This technology is based on the ability of visible or ultraviolet light to interact with light-sensitive compounds (photoinitiators) in the gel matrix to create free radicals that, in turn, initiate polymerization, forming crosslinked hydrogels. Advantages of this technique include better spatial and temporal control of polymerization, rapid cure rates, minimal heat production, and the ability to be synthesized in situ.[31] Although the relative paucity of nontoxic monomers and organic solvents usable for photopolymerization is a concern in in-vivo applications, certain applications have promise for clinical use. For example, polyvinyl alcohol hydrogels (used in ophthalmic materials and tendon repair), formed by conventional freeze-thaw, chemical aldehyde crosslinking, or radiation processes have traditionally created harsh environments not compatible with cellular and tissue viability. More recent photopolymerized polyvinyl alcohol hydrogels have, however, seeded human dermal fibroblasts in culture.[35] In-vivo applications will likely soon follow.

Growth Factors

Growth factors are soluble peptide gene products capable of binding cellular receptors and effectuating either a permissive or preventive response by the cell toward differentiation, proliferation, or both. Research into growth factors has blossomed over the last decade, with great strides being made in understanding the structure, expression, and function of these soluble mediators of cellular activity. Their precise role in tissue engineering and their enormous potential for therapeutic use are, however, only beginning to be understood.

Growth and differentiation of cells is generally understood to be influenced by the interplay of soluble growth factors with their environment, which includes the insoluble extracellular matrix, growth substrates, and mediators of cellular interaction. The impetus to tissue engineering research therefore becomes mimicking the spatial and temporal complexity of growth factor release and manipulating this release for therapeutic benefit in tissue regeneration and repair.

A recent review of the data on growth factors and their receptors, as well as extracellular matrix and adhesion molecules being investigated with regard to mesenchymal stem cells, begins to illustrate the tremendous promise of this research in the field of regenerative medicine.[9] Matrix molecules include, but are not limited to, collagen (type I–VI), proteoglycan, fibronectin, laminin, and hyaluronan. Adhesion molecules facilitating cellular-extracellular matrix contact fall into the category of integrins, whereas growth factors described to date include interleukins, transforming growth factor (TGF), tumor necrosis factor (TNF), colony stimulating factor (CSF), platelet derived growth factor (PDGF), insulin growth factor (IGF), and fibroblast growth factor (FGF). Clearly, adequate discussions of these molecules extend beyond the scope of this chapter. For our purposes, it is sufficed to review the core principles of molecular signaling before discussing applications in tissue engineering.

Cellular morphology, signaling, and ultimately survival in large part are mediated by adhesion mechanisms between cells and the underlying substrates or extracellular matrix. A key player in this interaction is the family of integrins; transmembrane receptor glycoproteins made up of alpha and beta subunits involved in cell-cell and cell-extracellular matrix adhesion, leading to the initiation of intracellular signaling mechanisms. For example, integrin-mediated adhesion leads to rapid recruitment and activation of numerous secondary messengers, including focal adhesion kinase (FAK), mitogen-activated protein kinase (MAPK), and phospholipase-C gamma (PLC-gamma). Focal adhesion kinase activation leads to the formation of a FAK-Src complex that is central to regulating the downstream signaling pathways that control cellular spreading, movement, and survival.[36] Mitogen-activated protein kinase controls proliferation, differentiation, and apoptotic signaling pathways, whereas phospholipase C gamma is involved in growth-factor-induced calcium release by cells, as well as in signaling calcium entry across cellular membranes.[37,38]

Emerging research reveals that signaling between growth factors and extracellular matrix molecules may be synergistic. For example, integrin and growth-factor-mediated responses are regulated by common intracellular signaling pathways, including MAPK and PLC.[39] Although the exact relationship between pathway activation and the extent and direction of cellular growth and differentiation remains unclear, several studies have found potential therapeutic benefit by manipulating this pathway. For example, fibrin used as a dermal substrate to culture skin substitutes increases vascular endothelial growth factor secretion, which in turn improves regeneration of epidermal structures after in-vivo transplantation. It also improves the vascularity of the construct by promoting migration of vascular endothelial cells.[40] Transforming growth factor beta-1 (TGF-beta1), PDGF, and FGF have additive effects on ligamentous regeneration and repair in vitro when cultured in collagen-glycosaminoglycan scaffolds.[41]

Syncronism Toward Tissue Engineering Constructs

Thus far, the discussions of stem-cell, polymer, and growth-factor research have been made in relative isolation from one another; however, the enormous potential of these techniques in combination to create new treatment options in regenerative medicine should be obvious. For example, chondrocytes can induce cellular de-differentiation into a proliferative state, followed by re-differentiation to mature matrix-secreting forms in vitro by sequential administration of selected growth factors.[42] Hydrogels can provide controlled release of select growth factors useful in cartilage engineering.[43] The interplay between these tissue engineering techniques will undoubtedly lead to novel therapeutic applications.

The Future of Tissue Engineering

Over the past decade, investment in tissue engineering research is estimated to be more than $600 million annually, representing a 16% growth rate and more than $3.5 billion in aggregate investment.[44] Structural applications (development of skeletal tissues) are the fastest growing segment, with stem-cell research programs spearheading the way. In the United States, most funding has been for commercial development, whereas in Japan and Europe, governmental funding has included more basic research.[45] Laboratories outside the United States

have traditionally enjoyed more freedom from regulatory constraints; however, this situation may be changing with the appearance of autogenic replacement options. Quality control standard for the release of final products remain to be established because traditional double-blinded, placebo-controlled studies and animal models do not reliably predict human outcomes.[46]

Regardless of present bureaucratic limitations, tissue engineering continues to progress rapidly and is poised to make tremendous contributions to the treatment of innate and acquired disease.

References

1. Yannas IV. The missing organ and how to replace it. In: *Tissue and Organ Regeneration in Adults*. Yannas, IV, author. New York: Springer-Verlag, 2001.
2. Walgenbach KJ, Voigt M, Riabikhin AW, et al. Tissue engineering in plastic reconstructive surgery. *Anatomic Rec.* 2001;263:372–378.
3. Vats S, Tolley NS, Polak J., et al. Stem cells: sources and applications. *Clin Otolaryngol.* 2002;27:227–232.
4. Thompson JA, Itskovitz-Eldor J, Shapiro SS. Embryonic stem cells derived from human blastocysts. *Science.* 1998;282:1142–1145.
5. Matsui Y, Zsebo K, Hogan BL. Derivation of pluripotent embryonic stem cells from murine primordial germ cells in culture. *Cell.* 1002;70:841–847.
6. Henningson CT, Stanislaus MA, Gerwirtz AM. Embryonic and adult stem cell therapy. *J Allergy Clin Immunol.* 2003;111:S745–753.
7. Korbling M, Estrov Z, Champlin R. Adult stem cells and tissue repair. Bone Marrow *Transplant.* 2003;32:S23–24.
8. Petersen BE, Terada N. Stem cells: a journey into a new frontier. *J Am Soc Nephrol.* 2001;12:1773–1780.
9. Ringe J, Kaps C, Burmester GR, Sittinger M. Stem cells for regenerative medicine: advances in the engineering of tissues and organs. *Naturwissenschaften.* 2002;89:338–351.
10. Caplan AI, Bruder SP. Mesenchymal stem cells: building blocks for molecular medicine in the 21th century. *Trends Molec Med.* 2001;7:259–265.
11. Passier R, Mummery C. Origin and use of embryonic and adult stem cells in differentiation and tissue repair. *Cardiovasc Res.* 2003;58:324–335.
12. Drukker M, Katz G, Urbach A. Characterization of the expression of MHC proteins in human embryonic stem cells. *Proc Natl Acad Sci USA.* 2002;99:9864–9869.
13. Watt FM, Hogan BL. Out of Eden: stem cells and their niches. *Science.* 200;287:1427–1430.
14. Mahoney MJ, Saltzman WM. Transplantation of brain cells assembled around a programmable synthetic microenvironment. *Nature Biotech.* 2001;19:934–939.
15. Breuls RGM, Mol A, Petterson R, Oomens CWJ, Baaijens FPT, Bouten CVC. Monitoring local cell viability in engineered tissues: a fast, quantitative and non destructive approach. *Tissue Eng.* 2003;9:269–281.
16. Piskin E. Biodegradable polymeric matrices for bio-artificial implants. *Int J Artif Organ.* 2002;25:434–440.

17. Benya PD, Scaffer JD. Dedifferentiated chondrocytes re-express the differentiated collagen phenotype when cultured in agarose gels. *Cell.* 1982;30:215–224.

18. Hollister SJ, Maddox RD Taboas JM. Optimal design and fabrication of scaffolds to mimic tissue properties and satisfy biological constraints. *Biomaterials.* 2002; 23:4095–4103.

19. Lu L, Zhu X, Valenzuela RG, Currier BL, Yaszemski MJ. Biodegradable polymer scaffolds for cartilage tissue engineering. *Clin Orthop Rel Res.* 2001;391S:S251–270.

20. Voytik-harbin SL, Roeder BA, Sturgis JE, Kokini K, Robinson JP. Simultaneous mechanical loading and confocal reflection microscopy for three-dimensional microbiomechanical analysis of biomaterials and tissue constructs. *Microscop Microanal.* 2003;9:74–85.

21. Marques AP, Reis RL, Hunt JA. The biocompatibility of novel starch-based polymers and composites: in-vitro studies. *Biomaterials.* 2002;23:1471–1478.

22. Zhang Y, Ni M, Zhang M, Ratner B. Calcium phosphate-chitosan composite scaffolds for bone tissue engineering. *Tissue Eng.* 2003;9:337–345.

23. Kast CE, Frick W, Losert U, Bernkop-Schnurch A. Chitosan-thioglycolic acid conjugate: a new scaffold material for tissue engineering? *Int J Pharma.* 2003;256:183–189.

24. Gentleman E, Lay AN, Dickerson DA, Nauman EA, Livesay GA, Dee KC. Mechanical characterization of collagen fibers and scaffolds for tissue engineering. *Biomaterials.* 2003;24:3805–3813.

25. Pieper JS, Van Der Kraan PM, et al. Crosslinked type II collagen matrices: preparation, characterization and potential for cartilage engineering. *Biomaterials.* 2002;23:3183–3192.

26. Sachlos E, Reis N, Ainsley C, Derby B, Czernuszka JT. Novel collagen scaffolds with predefined internal morphology made by solid freeform fabrication. *Biomaterials.* 2003;24:1487–1497.

27. Griffith LG. Emerging design principles in biomaterials and scaffolds for tissue engineering. *Ann NY Acad Sci.* 2002;961:83–95.

28. Wang YC, Lin MC, Wang DM, Hsieh HJ. Fabrication of a novel porous PGA chitosan hybrid matrix for tissue engineering. *Biomaterials.* 2003;24:1047–1057.

29. Leonor IB, Ito A, Onuma K, Kanzaki N, Reis RL. In vitro bioactivity of starch thermoplastic/hydroxyapatite composite biomaterials: an in situ study using atomic force microscopy. *Biomaterials.* 2003;24:579–585.

30. Gutowska A, Jeong B, Jasionowski M. Injectable gels for tissue engineering. *Anatom Rec.* 2001;263:342–349.

31. Nguyen KT, West JL. Photopolymerizable hydrogels for tissue engineering applications. *Biomaterials.* 2002; 23:4307–14.

32. Cao YL, Ibarra C, Vacanti C. Preparation and Use of Thermosensitive Polymers. In: *Tissue Engineering: Methods and Protocols.* Totowa NJ: Humana Press, 1999.

33. Vacanti CA, Langer R, Schloo B, Vacanti JP. Synthetic polymers seeded with chondrocytes provide a template for new cartilage formation. *Plast Reconst Surg.* 1991;95:843–850.

34. Lutolf MP, Lauer-Fields JL, Schmoekel HG, et al. Synthetic matrix mettaloproteinse-sensitive hydrogels for the conduction of tissue regeneration: engineering cell-invasion characteristics. *Proc Nat Acad Sci.* 2003;100:5413–548.

35. Schmedlen RH, Masters KS, West JL. Photocrosslinkable polyvinyl alcohol hydrogels that can be modified with cell adhesion peptides for use in tissue engineering. *Biomaterials.* 2002;23:4325–4332.

36. Parsons JT, Martin KH, Slack JK, Taylor, JM, Weed SA. Focal adhesion kinase: a regulator of focal adhesion dynamics and cell movement. *Oncogene.* 2000;19:5606–5613.

37. Robinson MJ, Cobb MH. Mitogen-activated protein kinase pathways. *Curr Opin Cell Biol.* 1997;9:180–186.

38. Putney JW. PLC-gamma: an old player has a new role. *Nat Cell Biol.* 2002;4:E280–281.

39. Bottaro DP, Liebmann-Vinson A, Heidaran MA. Molecular signaling in bioengineered tissue microenviron ments. *Ann NY Acad Sci.* 2002;961:143–153.

40. Hojo S, Inokuchi S, Kidokoro M, et al. Induction of vascular endothelial growth factor by fibrin as a dermal substrate for cultured skin substitute. *Plast Reconst Surg.* 2003;111:1638–1645.

41. Meaney Murray M, Rice K, Wright RJ, Spector M. The effect of selected growth factors on human anterior cruciate ligament cell interactions with a three-dimensional collagen GAG scaffold. *J Orthop Res.* 2003;2:238–244.

42. Pei M, Seidel J, Vunjak-Novakovic G, Freed LE. Growth factors for sequential cellular de- and re-differentiation in tissue engineering. *Biochem Biophys Res Com.* 2002;294:149–154.

43. Elisseeff J, McIntosh W, Fu K, Blunk BT, Langer R. Controlled-release of IGF-1 and TGF-beta1 in a photopolymerizing hydrogel for cartilage tissue engineering. *J Orthop Res.* 2001;19:1098–1104.

44. Lysaght MJ, Reyes J. The growth of tissue engineering. *Tissue Eng.* 2001;7:485–490.

45. McIntire LV. World technology panel report on tissue engineering. *Ann Biomed Eng.* 2002;30:1216–1220.

46. Naughton GK. From lab bench to market: critical issues in tissue engineering. *Ann NY Acad Sci.* 2002;961:372–385.

12

The Role of Stem Cells in Plastic Surgery

Maria Z. Siemionow and Selahattin Özmen

Introduction

Stem cell transplantation has become an increasingly important treatment for a wide variety of onco-hematological and metabolic disorders. Improvement in the therapeutic supplementation has reduced the incidence of severe and fatal side effects; however, complications still need to be minimized.

In 1949 Jacobsen et al.[1] and in 1951 Lorenz et al.[2] first raised the possibility of injecting bone marrow intravenously to rescue lethally irradiated animals. In 1961, Till and McCulloch showed that spleen-derived hematopoietic stem cells (HSC) were able to reconstitute radiation-induced hematopoietic failure in mice.[3] At that time, HSCs were believed to:

- Have the capacity for radioprotection
- Be able to develop cells of all hematopoietic lineages
- Have the capacity for self-renewal

Soon it became clear that HSCs were only a fraction of hematopoietic cells and that they could be harvested from the spleen or bone marrow.

Hematopoietic cells were subfractionated based on size, density, and the expression of certain cell surface markers.[4] Approximately 1 in 2,000 marrow cells (0.05%) is a HSC.[5]

CD34 is a transmembrane cell surface sialomucin present on 1% to 4% of stem cells and their progeny[5] and on vascular endothelial cells.[6] More than 90% of CD34+ cells express antigens that are characteristic of commitment to the lymphoid, myeloid, or erythroid lineages, and, therefore, are not considered stem cells with pluripotent reconstitutive potential.[7] Cells that initiate long-term marrow cultures, "long-term culture initiating cells [LTC-IC]", express CD34 and do not express lineage antigens such as CD3, CD4, CD8, CD10, CD14, CD15, CD19, CD20, CD33, CD38, and CD71 (CD34+ Lin– cells). The HSC is currently defined and used as CD34+ DR–Lin–.

Cell surface molecules that appear to be useful in selecting primitive and multipotential stem cells against committed progenitor cells include CD38, HLA class II (DR) antigens, and Thy-1 (CDw90). Only 1% of the CD34+ cells do not express the CD38 antigen.[8] These CD34+ CD38– cells appear as homogenous primitive blast cells with self-renewing potential. A sufficient number of early and pluripotent hematopoietic progenitor cells with indefinite self-renewal potential is required for complete and constant hematopoietic engraftment after myeloablative therapy. In humans, the minimum number of early progenitor cells that will supply complete and permanent engraftment has not yet been determined.

Sources of Hematopoietic Stem Cells

Hematopoietic stem cells come from bone marrow, fetal liver cells, peripheral blood stem cells (PBSC), embryonic stem cells, umbilical cord blood, and in-vitro expansion of stem cells.

Hematopoietic Stem Cells From Bone Marrow

The traditional method of stem cell transplantation was to infuse an unmanipulated, complete mixture of marrow cells. A fairly large amount of cells was infused: amounts in the range of 0.4 to 1.2×10^8 mononuclear cells (MNC)/kg body weight are required for a stem cell transplant with a complete marrow cell suspension.[9] A stem cell transplant with complete marrow yielded a lower rate of graft failure and a substantially lower relapse rate.

The marrow suspension consists of a complex heterogeneity of cells, including the essential population of HSCs. As in the case of an allogeneic transplant, the increased dissimilarity between donor and recipient would cause severe side effects, such as graft-versus-host-disease. Depletion of the proportion of marrow T cells considerably reduces the frequency and severity of GVHD but also occasionally causes poor engraftment.[10]

Hematopoietic Stem Cells From Fetal Liver Cells

From the second to the seventh months of pregnancy, the liver of the fetus is physiologically a part of the hematopoietic tissues. Fetal liver cells can reconstitute successfully both hematopoietic and lymphopoietic systems, and they could be used for transplantation before the onset of lymphopoiesis.[11]

Hematopoietic Stem Cells From Peripheral Blood

Bone marrow and peripheral blood stem-cell (PBSC) pools maintain a dynamic equilibrium, allowing hematopoietic progenitor cells migrating from extravascular marrow sites into circulation and vice versa. The number of steady-state progenitor cells circulating in the peripheral blood at any given time is usually too low for a safe transplant dose.[12]

The clinical use of PBSCs has expanded rapidly since the first report detailing their use was published in 1981. Peripheral blood stem cells largely replaced bone marrow as the preferred stem cell source largely as a result of quicker engraftment kinetics and ease of collection. The number of CD34+ cells collected by apheresis from one donor can exceed the CD34+ cells contained in a bone marrow graft by fourfold.[13] The use of PBSCs in allogeneic transplantation has also increased greatly.

The possibility of harvesting progenitor cells by leukapheresis was first demonstrated in 1980.[14] Clinical studies about successful blood progenitor cell mobilization and reports of the advantage of mobilized blood cells in the hematopoietic reconstition soon followed.

Peripheral blood stem cells have several advantages when compared to marrow grafts:

1. Collecting stem cells does not require hospital admission or exposure to general anesthesia.

2. PBSCs have a shorter period of cytopenia after myeloablative therapy than do cells from marrow. Both neutrophils and platelets are recovered much more rapidly with growth-factor mobilized PBSCs than with marrow cells. Bone marrow has the highest percentage of CD34+ MNC per milliliter; however, an even higher absolute number of CD34+ cells can be collected from peripheral blood after mobilization with chemotherapy and growth factor.

3. Peripheral blood is less likely than marrow to contain malignant cells.

4. Mononuclear cells collected during leukapheresis contain colony-forming unit granulocyte macrophage (CFU-GM) and CD34+ cells,[15] which can be isolated and cryopreserved.

Mobilization Protocols

Within the marrow microenvironment, the majority of CD34– stem cells are stationary while they rest. Some of these stem cells circulate in the peripheral blood, and they can still return to bone marrow and down-regulate CD34– expression. In normal conditions, few activated progenitor cells respond to growth factor-mediated signals. In some conditions, the number of peripheral cycling stem cell increases[16]:

Myelosuppressive Chemotherapy. During recovery from myelosuppressive chemotherapy, the number of PB CFU-GM cells increases by 50-fold.[17] High-dose cyclophosphamides are most often used for mobilization. However, chemotherapy mobilization has some limitations, such as neutropenic sepsis, bleeding diathesis, and the unpredictability of the timing of apheresis.

Myelosuppressive Chemotherapy Plus Hematopoietic Growth Factors. When G-CSF or GM-CSF is given after chemotherapy, the concentration of progenitors in the peripheral blood is amplified, allowing more progenitors to be collected with fewer phresis procedures. The addition of these growth factors to myelosuppressive chemotherapy also enhances mobilization and reduces myelotoxicity. The amplitude of the circulating stem cell concentration is related to the intensity of the myelosuppressive agents used.[18]

Hematopoietic Growth Factors Alone for Collection of PBSCs. Hematopoietic growth factors alone are often used to mobilize hematopoietic progenitor cells. The exact mechanism of colony stimulating factor (CSF)-depended mobilization is not known. CSFs may release the stem cells from marrow into blood. HSCs increase several days after initiation of therapy; therefore, cytokines probably act by stimulating the proliferation of stem cells, either directly or by a secondary release of endogenous cytokines by stromal cells. Some of the factors used to mobilize HSC are G-CSF, G-CSF/SCF, GM-CSF, IL-3, Flt3 ligand alone or with G-CSF/GM-CSF, PIXY321 (IL 3, GM-CSF fusion protein), human erythropoietin, and IL-6, IL-1, and IL-8.

Factors Affecting Yield

There are several factors that affect progenitor cell mobilization after myelosuppressive chemotherapy:

1. Previous wide-field radiotherapy
2. The severity of myelosuppression and the rate of leukocyte recovery
3. The duration of previous chemotherapy
4. The number of cycles of chemotherapy
5. The interval between previous chemotherapy and mobilization
6. Exposure to drugs toxic to stem cells, such as BCNU and melphalan
7. The addition of G-CSF or GM-CSF to myelosuppressive chemotherapy

Techniques of Collection

Optimal Time for Peripheral Blood Stem Cell Collection. Collecting sufficient progenitor cells for rescue from a single apheresis is a goal for many authors. Timing PBSC collection properly is important to maximize the number of progenitors harvested. However, the most reliable time for harvesting hematopoietic stem cells has yet to be determined. In current protocols, pheresis is usually initiated 10 to 18 days after

the administration of low-to-moderate-dose chemotherapy[16] or when the leukocyte count rises above 1×10^9/L and continues until an arbitrary target, such as $3, \times 10^8$ mononuclear cells/kg BW, is reached.[19] However, different WBC counts are used for collection by different authors.

The main indicator of HSCs with reconstitutive potential in apheresis products is CFU-GM. Also, monitoring daily CD34+ cell count in the peripheral blood may help predict the best time for leukapheresis. Colony Forming Unit (CFU) assays are time-consuming and difficult to standardize. Counting CD34+ cells may be preferable because it is a more direct measure of progenitor cells. The minimal CD34+ cell dose required in the autologous transplant is suggested to be around 1×10^6/kg.[20] However, recovery is faster with higher CD34+ cell doses, and different centers recommend levels between 2×10^6/kg and 5×10^6/kg as the safe engrafting dose. Thus, the best time to begin apheresis after chemotherapy requires further study.

Target and Thresholds. The number of progenitor cells infused directly affects hematopoietic reconstitution. Effective hematopoietic reconstitution requires a progenitor cell dose above the minimum threshold. Unlike the situation with bone marrow transplantation, the dose of nucleated cells does not appear to predict hematopoietic reconstitution as well as the dose of progenitor cells.[21]

Another variable important in determining the progenitor cell threshold for rapid engraftment is previous chemotherapy. Prolonged chemotherapy may reduce the quality of CD34+ cells or cause concomitant stromal damage, interfering with engraftment.

Identifying PBSCs. Peripheral blood stem cells are CD34+ /CD38– Thy-1 and do not express a full complement of either myeloid or lymphoid lineage-specific markers (Lin–).[22] PBSCs are neither phenotypically nor immunologically identical to bone marrow derived stem cells. Mobilized PBSCs are less active in cellular cycling (they have a lower proportion of cells in S phase), express more lineage-specific differentiation antigens, and are less metabolically active.[23] Furthermore, PBSCs have higher clonogenicity in long-term culture assays.

Some authors suggest that transplanting PBSCs instead of marrow may result in faster engraftment and improved immune reconstitution.[23] Despite the fact that PBSC grafts contain more donor T lymphocytes than do marrow grafts, which is a possible cause of both acute and chronic GVHD, the incidence of acute GVHD after PBSC is no higher than that with marrow transplantation.[24] However, the incidence of chronic GVHD in PBSC transplantation may be higher.[25] Therefore, at present, allogeneic PBSC transplantation should not be routinely performed instead of marrow transplantation.

Mobilization and Collection of PBSCs

Continuous-Flow Stem Cell Apheresis. Peripheral blood stem cells are collected by single or multiple, continuous-flow apheresis, generally through peripheral venous access, although occasionally central venous access is required.[26] Between 2 and 3.5 times the donor's blood volume is processed per run; however, up to 6 times the donor's blood volume processing has been reported.[27] Stem cells and granulocytes are separated from the red blood cell and plasma fractions by centrifugation, and the latter two components are returned to the donor.

ACD-A, alone or in combination with heparin, is used for anticoagulation, and calcium replacement is required when ACD-A alone is used in large-volume leukapheresis.

For allogeneic transplantation, cells are either frozen or transfused fresh. Cryopreserved stem cells have the advantage of being harvested independently of the time they are transplanted to the patient. Also, alloreactive, GVHD-inducing cells may be lost selectively by the cryopreservation and defrosting procedures.

Collecting Stem Cells from Normal Donors. Syngeneic or allogeneic transplants using PBSC are uncommon as a result of the concern about donor toxicities from growth factor administration and the theoretically increased risk of GVHD from the large number of allografted T cells.[28]

Although most donors experience bone pain and headache, mobilizing HSC by rHuG-CSF is safe in normal donors, and serious adverse effects are rare.[29] However, even in healthy donors vary widely in their ability to mobilize PBSCs. No increase in acute GVHD compared to marrow

has been reported in preliminary studies of allogeneic PBSC transplantation.[5] These results suggest that PBSCs will likely be used for the majority of allogeneic and autologous transplants in the near future.

There are a number of unanswered questions about progenitor cell mobilization[29]:

- What cytokine regimen is optimal?
- How do different mobilization regimens affect the quality of the PBPC graft?
- Can the efficacy of stem cell mobilization be predicted (PB CD34+ cell concentration at steady-state, adhesion molecules, and so on)?

Engraftment and Kinetics

The recovery of hematopoiesis is more rapid after transplantation of mobilized PBPCs than after transplantation of bone marrow.[30] This difference could be the result of a larger progenitor cell dose or of a higher percentage of late, lineage-committed progenitor cells in the apheresis product, requiring less time to transit cell-differentiating compartments.

In PBSC transplantation, doses lower than 2×10^6 cells/kg of recipient body weight are reported to be associated with prolonged cytopenias and increased early mortality.[31] Higher doses of CD34+ cells may lead to quicker engraftment, especially with greatly increased doses.[31] However, an obligate period of profound pancytopenia, lasting approximately 8 days would be seen, despite transplantation of maximal cell doses, including progenitor cells.[29]

Increased rates of GVHD have been seen in PBSC transplants enriched by in-vitro CD34+ cell selection; alterations in the cytokine expression patterns of transplanted cells or changes in lymphocyte subsets delivered with the graft might be possible factors in this increase.[32] T-cell depletion of the grafts leads to lower rates of GVHD; however, a slightly higher incidence of graft rejection would occur.

Combined PBSC and bone marrow transplants can also shorten the time to engraftment. Primarily because of the use of recombinant human hematopoietic growth factors, the costs of stem cell mobilization and collection are greater for PBSC than for bone marrow transplantation.

Benefits and Drawbacks of PBPC Transplantation

Shorter hospitalization from more rapid hematopoietic recovery (thus fewer days at risk for infection), reduces the overall morbidity and cost of PBPC transplantation. The cost effectiveness of the procedure primarily depends on the costs of chemopriming, growth factors, and the number of aphereses needed. Establishment of an unrelated PBPC donor program, similar to the National Marrow Donor Program, is being discussed. Such a program would reach far more potential stem cell donors and offer greater access to minorities.

Disadvantages of PBPC transplantation include the following[33]:

1. The need for vascular access
2. The chemopriming for HSC mobilization
3. The adverse effects of cytokine treatment
4. The variability of HSC mobilization efficiency
5. The induced leukocytes

In about 80% of cases, some minor side effects of growth factors were seen, such as headache, fever, bone pain, and myalgias. Administration of rHuG-CSF is safer in healthy donors. Important morbidities, including splenic rupture and death, have rarely been reported.

Allogeneic Transplantation of PBSCs

There was initial caution about allogeneic blood cell transplantation because of the potential of severe GVHD from the high number of T cells infused and the uncertainty about the safety of administering recombinant growth factor for mobilization.

In PBPC allotransplants, compared to bone marrow allografts, the average number of CD34+ cells is 4 times higher and the number of T cells and natural killer cells is 10 to 20 times higher.[23] Although these results lead to concerns that PBPC allotransplants could produce more severe GVHD, rapid engraftment and increase in rates of acute GVHD have been reported.[34]

In conclusion, only a single trial has reported a higher incidence of acute GVHD after PBSC than after traditional bone marrow transplantation.[24]

Some important points of allogeneic blood cell transplantation[35]:

- The lower number of T cells infused may enable less-intensive GVHD prophylaxis.
- Allogeneic hematopoietic progenitor cells provide a tumor-free graft with possible graft-versus-tumor activity.
- The avoidance of general anesthesia and trauma to soft tissue and bone more than compensates for the potential risk of G-CSF administration.
- Persistent long-term engraftment beyond 2 years has been shown[23] with no report of late graft failure.
- After mobilized blood cell transplants, naive and memory helper T-cell and B- cell recovery is more rapid than bone marrow transplants. As a result, allogeneic PBSC transplants are promising and do not appear to increase the risk of acute GVHD in preliminary studies, but further follow-up is necessary for evaluation of chronic GVHD.

Conclusions About PBSC Transplantation

Hematopoietic stem cell peripheralization allows collection of large doses of progenitors and avoids multiple bone marrow aspirations and the need for general anesthesia. PBPC transplantation provides rapid hematological recovery and, in most studies, has reduced hospitalization and costs. The optimal dose of cells, the means of mobilization, and the cellular composition of the stem cell graft need to be further investigated. In conclusion, PBPC transplantation is as effective as bone marrow transplantation as a source of HSC. Initial data with PBSC allotransplants justify further evaluation. In the long-term, it is likely the PBPCs will replace bone marrow as the preferred source of hematopoietic cells for transplantation.

Hematopoietic Stem Cells From Embryonic Stem Cells

Embryonic stem cells (ESCs) are totipotent cells isolated from the inner cell mass of blastocysts. They can give rise to every cell in the mature organism.[36] Throughout development from blastocyst to fetus, totipotent stem cells loss their totipotency, which is replaced by a limited programming toward endoderm, mesoderm, or ectoderm, and at last single-tissue specificity. Totipotent stem cells can produce cells that originate from all three germ layers but not those from the extraembryonic structures; thus, they cannot form the complete embryo.

Several soluble factors direct the differentiation of mouse ESCs; for example, IL-6 directs cells to the erythroid lineage[37]; IL-3 directs cells to become macrophages, mast cells, or neutrophils[38]; and retinoic acid induces neuron formation.[39] None of the growth factors directs differentiation particularly to one cell type. Most of the growth factors are thought to inhibit differentiation of specific cell types, and this inhibitory effect is more evident than an induction effect.

Growth factors can be classified into 3 categories with respect to their overall effects:

1. Growth factors that mainly induce mesodermal cells; activin-A and TGF-_1.

2. Growth factors that activate ectodermal and mesodermal markers, such as retinoic acid, EGF, BMP-4, and bFGF.

3. Growth factors that allow differentiation into the three embryonic germ layers, NGF, and HGF.

Thus, certain classes of growth factors effect differentiation of specific germ layers.

Given their totipotency, ESCs may have potential uses in regenerative medicine.[40] Some reports indicate that mouse ESCs can be induced to differentiate into particular types of cells, including hematopoietic cells,[41] neurons,[42] cardiomyocytes,[43] and myocytes.[44] The exact mechanisms in the differentiation of the ESCs to this wide range of cell types are not clear, but the local environment is believed to be important.

Theoretically, ESCs can be maintained in an undifferentiated state indefinitely in vitro and directed to differentiate into any cell type of the body. This potential could supply some laboratory-produced artificial tissues—or even organs—to treat many diseases. On the other hand, although it has been more than 2 decades since murine ESCs were first isolated, ESC technology in humans is still in its infancy.

A number of obstacles must be overcome before ESCs can be applied clinically[45]: a gating procedure is needed to carefully select and to expand a pure population of the desired cell type; religious and moral concerns about the use of ESCs need to be addressed; and induction of the donor specific tolerance in the recipient is required for allogeneic transplantations.

The first step in an embryonic stem cell-based therapy is to establish ESCs that are capable of differentiating to a specific cell type and to purify this lineage from the mixed population. So far, no approach to the differentiation of ESCs has yet yielded a 100% pure population of mature progeny. For clinical applications, a simple genetic approach is needed for the production and proliferation of either pure populations of specific cell types, or cells that express suicidal genes to ablate the misbehaving cells. Implanting undifferentiated ESCs or inappropriate cell lineages carries the risk of teratoma formation or further perturbation of tissue function. Therefore, many basic questions regarding the biology of stem cells must be answered to overcome these difficulties.

Another equally challenging question that must be resolved is one of law, ethics, and some moral and religious concerns about human ESC use.

Finally, as with all allogeneic transplants, there is a risk of transplant rejection by the host. On the other hand, the ESC-derived cell transplant could be free of highly immunogenic mature dendritic cells and will express only major histocompatibility complex (MHC) class I, but not class II, at the time of transplantation. Because long-term maintenance of immunosuppressive therapy would limit successful clinical application, the creation of immune tolerance would enable the use of ESC-derived therapy.

Human ESC-based therapies are entirely novel, and serious concerns about safety and efficacy will need to be addressed before human clinical trials can be initiated.

Hematopoietic Stem Cells From Umbilical Cord Blood

Hematopoietic stem cells reach the blood and circulate throughout their development as well as during the perinatal shift of the sites for hematopoiesis. The possibility that HSCs from umbilical cord blood (UCB) could increase engraftment and decrease the incidence of GVHD has recently focused much attention on UCB. Assessing UCB at the time of birth without affecting the fetus or the mother is highly advantageous.

Several authors have reported that UCB might be an enriched source of HSCs. In clinical trials, UCB stem cell transplantation shows a high engraftment potential with a low risk of acute GVHD.[46] The absence of risks for the donor and a low risk of infectious disease transmission are advantages of UCB stem cell transplantation.[46] Because every newborn is a potential donor, UCB banking might theoretically provide a ready-to-use HSC source for every HLA type.

The main disadvantage of UCB is that the amount of blood that can be collected from a single donor is limited, and collection is a one-time-only procedure.

With refined techniques, up to 200 ml of UCB can be obtained, and it can contain as many as 4×10^6 myeloid progenitors; however, reported UCB volumes vary widely,[47] and recovering only 20 mL to 40 mL is not infrequent.[48]

Some obstetric factors may influence the final collection yield, such as the length of gestation, cord length, cord clamping position, time from infant delivery to cord clamping, infant weight, and level of the infant in relation to the placenta before and at the time of cord clamping.[49] The procedure followed and equipment used in collecting can also effect the final yield.

To date, there is no commercial system for the placenta suspension and manipulation. Open and closed collection systems have been described.[50–51] While the placenta is still in-utero, or just after placental delivery, open systems drain the blood from the maternal end of the severed cord into jars or tubes, and closed systems drain the blood by venipuncture using collection bags or syringes.[50] Umbilical cord blood for clinical use is usually collected after placenta delivery using a closed system to prevent bacterial and maternal blood contamination and to avoid interferences with the delivery procedure.[51]

An ideal collection system should meet the following criteria[51]:

1. It should allow an easy, quick, and suitable positioning of the placenta.
2. It should reduce the need of repositioning the placenta during collection.
3. It should "massage" the placenta to increase blood flow from the placenta to the umbilical vein.
4. It should minimize operator and environment contamination from potentially infected blood.
5. It should minimize the time and effort necessary to clean the collection area and to prepare for a new collection.

In conclusion, optimizing UCB collection procedures, together with improved HSC ex-vivo expansion techniques, may increase the clinical benefits of UCB. Using cryopreservation, UCB stem cells may be used for transplants in even older siblings or as target cells for a gene transfer.[52]

In-Vitro Expansion of the Hematopoietic Stem Cells

In-vitro expansion of progenitor and postprogenitor cells will reduce the need for leukapheresis and may expand an apheresis product with a low number of progenitor cells to provide sufficient cells.

Molecular engineering of cells is a new technology that is receiving much attention. Stem cells are attractive targets for molecular engineering because they have some desirable properties.[53]

- Gene transfer into HSCs would lead to a continuous supply of genetically modified hematopoietic cells. HSCs could provide a lifelong source of amplified progeny expressing the introduced gene.
- Potential viral vectors, especially retroviruses, can enter and be integrated with the DNA of early hematopoietic progenitor cells.
- Successful allogeneic bone marrow transplantation can correct several diseases of blood and immune cells, and these diseases could potentially be treated by expression of wild type genes in hematopoietic stem cells.
- Many inherited enzyme deficiency diseases can be treated by circulating the multiple lineages of HSC-derived blood and immune cells through the entire organism.

Retroviral vectors can reliably integrate genes efficiently into the genome of target cells. Packaging cells, which allow the production of replication-defective recombinant virus, free of wild-type virus, can provide efficient and safe retrovirus-mediated gene transfer.[54] Also, the adeno-associated viruses can be used to transfer genes into target cells. Adenoviruses allow the production of high virion titers, stabilize recombinant virions without helper contamination, and have potentially better safety characteristics.[55]

Gene therapy has several disadvantages. Stem cell capability can be easily lost during in vitro manipulation; poor engraftment from cultured stem cells has been reported.[56] Moreover, hematopoietic progenitor cells from bone marrow lose their stem cell ability more easily than HSCs in peripheral blood.[57] Therefore, the difference between stem cells at different stages of development should be considered when designing therapeutic strategies, including ex vivo manipulation of HSCs.[58]

Low gene transfer efficiency is still a challenge for human HSCs. The self-renewal frequency of murine HSCs is higher than it is in larger animals, so that the cells are expected to divide at least once during a few days of a standard retroviral transduction period. However, in larger animals, the frequency of self-renewal of HSCs may be much lower.[59] During a transduction period, even in the presence of hematopoietic cytokines, these cells unlikely cycle, and may differentiate or lose their engraftment capabilities. Also, human HSCs have far fewer retroviral receptors on their cell surfaces than do murine HSCs, which limits the transduction of human HSCs.[60]

Inducing differentiation in gene transfer experiments is important to get mature functional cells; however, differentiation can also be a problem because true stem cells have to be maintained in vitro. For increasing the rate of homologous recombination, new techniques are under development.

Recent Advances in Stem Cell Therapy

Our knowledge about stem cells is increasing at an incredible rate. By the time you read this chapter, there will most probably be some new and very important development about stem cells and their applications. The more we learn about stem cells, the more we understand their potential in medicine and in the field of reconstructive and aesthetic procedures.

Before describing the possible treatments offered by stem cells, we will consider two new members of the stem cell family: adult stem-progenitor cells and mesenchymal stem-progenitor cells. The importance of embryonic, peripheral blood and umbilical cord stem cells is well known, as described above. However, in recent years, adult stem cells have proved to have the ability to differentiate into multiple cell types, other than those of the tissue in which they reside. In-vitro expansion of adult and mesenchymal stem cells and using these cells in tissue engineering are very promising techniques for reconstructing different types of tissues.

Adult Stem Cells

Adult stem cells (ASCs) are a small fraction of the total number of cells in each tissue. An ACS is an undifferentiated cell that has the capability for self-renewal throughout its lifetime. In human adult bone marrow, they comprise between 1 in 10,000 and 1 in 100,000 or more of total blood cells.

Adult stem cells are identified by two main characteristics: cellular morphology and specific marker proteins linking them to the tissue or organ in which they exist. Until recently, human adult stem cells were thought to be developmentally committed and able to differentiate only into cell lineages from the tissue in which they resided. However, a number of experiments have showed that adult stem cells have the ability to differentiate into multiple cell types, an ability termed "plasticity" or "transdifferentiation" (Figure 12-1). Human ASC studies have shown differentiation into cardiac muscle cells[61]; skeletal myoblasts[62]; neuroectodermal lines, including brain cells of all types (neurons, oligodendrocytes, and astrocytes)[63]; hepatocytes and cholangiocytes[64]; epithelial cells of the skin, liver, digestive (esophageal, intestinal, gastric) and respiratory systems[65]; and endothelial cells.[66] Transdifferentiation studies are based on the idea that the particular environment determines the development of tissue-specific stem cells. Signals from a distant or adjacent tissue might delay these limiting signals and guide the cells to differentiate into particular tissues.[67]

Another important characteristic of ASCs is their capability to migrate from their niches to sites of tissue growth and repair. Bone marrow-derived stem cells migrate from bone marrow to differentiate and integrate into skin, lung, intestine, and stomach tissues.[65]

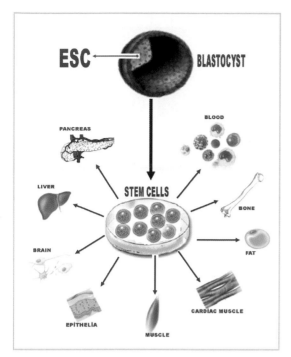

Figure 12 1. Plasticity of stem cells. Adult stem cells have the ability to differentiate into multiple cell types. (ESC: Embryonic stem cells from the inner surface of the blastocyst).

In theory, these cells could be differentiated in the laboratory and transplanted back into the same individual for tissue repair, thus bypassing the need for immunosuppression. However, for some stem cell types, difficulties in accessing the niche and isolating the cells, low frequency, poor growth in cell culture, and restricted lineage potential may make their use impractical for tissue engineering.[68]

Mesenchymal Stem Cells

The adult bone marrow stroma contains a subpopulation of nonhematopoietic cells known as "mesenchymal stem cells" or "mesenchymal progenitor cells" (MSCs). They are multipotent precursors that can develop either in vitro or in vivo into distinct mesenchymal tissues, including bone, cartilage, fat, tendon, muscle, and marrow stroma, which makes them an attractive cell source for tissue engineering studies.[69] They represent only about 0.01% to 0.001% of the marrow cells; however, because they adhere to glass and plastic, they can easily be separated from HSCs.[70] Mesenchymal stem cells are present in several

tissues during human development. They reside in the adult bone marrow, fat, muscle, skin, and in other tissues and in the fetal bone marrow and liver.[71] In addition to potential uses in tissue engineering and cell-based therapy,[72,73] MSCs can be transduced with different retroviral and other vectors and can be used for somatic gene therapies of systemic or local diseases.

Bone marrow stroma is the major source for MSCs in humans. Marrow from the iliac crest is thought to be most suitable for isolating MSCs.[74] However, the number of bone marrow MSCs substantially decreases with age; thus, alternative sources are necessary for autologous and allogenic use.[75] Umbilical cord blood is a rich source of stem and progenitor cells, and the results of immunophenotyping and morphological studies of cultured MSC-like cells from human umbilical cord vein suggest that these cells closely resemble cultured MSCs obtained from bone marrow and other sources.[71]

Stem and Progenitor Cells in Allogeneic Transplantation

Solid organ transplantation has become an almost ordinary treatment for end-stage organ failure. However, despite improved immunosuppressive regimens, current immunosuppressive drugs are far from ideal; chronic graft rejection cannot be prevented; and long-term survival of all grafts is limited. Chronic rejection is the major cause of late allograft loss.[72]

The lifelong use of immunosuppressive drugs is associated with numerous complications, including poor wound healing, opportunistic infections, drug-related toxicities, skin malignancies, low-grade lymphomas (called posttransplant lymphoproliferative disorders), and end-organ toxicity, including renal failure.[73]

Composite tissue allografts (CTAs) are a combination of skin, tendons, nerves, muscle, or bone and may be the next frontier in reconstructive surgery. Applying CTAs in humans is supposed to be a more difficult than organ transplantation because[76] some of these tissues, such as skin, are believed to be more antigenic than any component of an organ transplant and because intact bone marrow could be a component of the graft, supplying a constant source of donor antigens after transplant.

Prolonged CTA survival is achievable in animals using immunosuppressive drugs;[77] how-

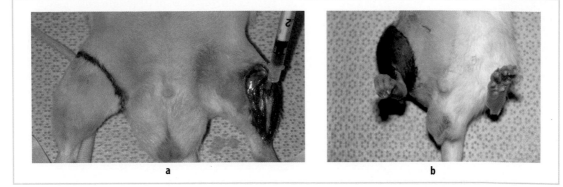

Figure 12-2. **a**) Intraosseous transplantation of the cellular bone-marrow-derived CD90+ stem and progenitor cells as a therapeutic approach to composite limb allograft transplantation. **b**) Limb allograft recipients at 7 days posttransplantation after treatment with CD90+ stem and progenitor cells without immunosuppression.

ever, using these drugs for non-life-threatening composite tissue reconstruction may not be clinically justified in humans. Creating donor-specific allograft tolerance would be the optimal approach for achieving permanent allograft survival by avoiding the need for long-term immunosuppressive treatment and preserving normal recipient immune function.[78]

Various attempts have been made to withdraw baseline immunosuppression regimens by inducing transplantation tolerance. One of the most effective and best-studied approaches to induce transplantation tolerance is bone marrow transplantation (BMT), which results in HSC chimerism. Bone marrow transplantation is thought to provide donor-specific, immune-tolerance induction by establishing mixed lymphoid chimerism.[79] Bone-marrow-transplantation-induced HSC macrochimerism can induce donor-specific tolerance to a variety of allografts in some experimental models.[80] We significantly

prolonged hind limb survival of rats using cellular and crude bone marrow delivery administered intraosseously. In a study of intraosseous (intratibial) cellular CD90+ stem cells transplantation, we prolonged the survival of the allogeneic rat hind limbs up to 15 days without immunosuppressive drug therapy (Figure 12-2).[81] In this study, flow cytometric analysis revealed a higher donor-specific chimerism level in the peripheral blood of the recipients from allograft treatment group (stem and progenitor cells injection) (Figure 12-3a) when compared with the chimerism level in the peripheral blood of the recipients from allograft control group no stem and progenitor cells treatment) (Figure 12-3b).

Using vascularized bone marrow transplantation in rat hind limb and rat vascularized groin skin/bone models, we prolonged allograft survival for more than 700 days under short-term (7-day) treatment with cyclosporine A and

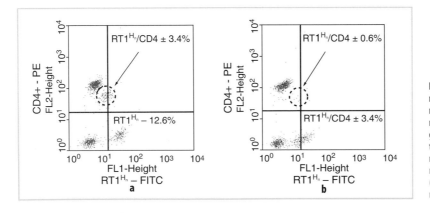

Figure 12-3. Flow cytometric analysis revealed a higher donor specific chimerism level in the peripheral blood of the recipients from a) allograft treatment group (stem and progenitor cells injection) when compared with b) the chimerism level in the peripheral blood of the recipients from allograft control group (no stem and progenitor cells treatment).

alpha-beta (α-β) T cell receptor monoclonal antibodies.[82]

Tolerance induction in allogeneic composite tissue transplantations using stem cell delivery is a promising approach and would allow the hand, larynx, tendons, nerves, and—even the face—to be transplanted without life-threatening immunosuppressive therapies.

Stem and Progenitor Cells in Tissue Engineering

Tissue engineering is a rapidly growing area since it became feasible to isolate living, healthy cells from the body, expand and combine them with biocompatible carrier materials, and retransplant them into patients.[67] Recently, much attention has been directed to multipotential embryonic, periosteal, and mesenchymal stem cells. The potential to differentiate stem cells into various tissues is important for regenerative medicine; however, we do not yet understand the differentiation processes and how to direct these cells to develop into the desired tissues. Early studies using bone marrow stromal cells for tissue repair focused on the repair of bone defects.[83] Some preclinical models, as well as clinical applications, currently being explored include keratinocytes or dermal fibroblasts for burn and wound repair,[84] chondrocytes for cartilage repair,[85] myocytes for myocardial repair,[86] retinal pigment epithelial cells for age-related macular degeneration,[87] and Schwann cell transplantation to restore myelin in CNS lesions.[88]

Tissue engineering using an individual's own bone marrow-derived MSCs to form implants in vitro is time consuming. Two alternatives are under investigation. The first is to prefabricate complex tissues with allogenic MSCs. Allogenic MSCs are used to generate tissue for transplant, which may be stored and implanted later. In large-animal models, donor-derived MSCs produced regenerative tissue similar to that produced by autologous MSCs.[67] Early studies showed that both animal and human MSCs do not express costimulatory antigens and, thus, seem to be immuno-privileged.[89]

The second alternative under investigation is direct in-vivo manipulation of the MSCs. A set of factors, which promotes chemoattraction of the MSCs, their site-specific mitotic expansion, their induction into and through a specific lineage, and the integration of the newly formed tissue within the host tissue, is needed for this approach.[89] It is possible to either inject or to immobilize these factors onto a scaffold before implantation.

Stem Cells in Bone Engineering

Reconstructing large bone segments is still a challenge. No approach suggested so far has proven to be ideal. Bone graft material, engineered with osteogenic committed cells combined with an osteoconductive scaffold, could be a promising approach. Some authors report good results in bone graft engineering using multipotent stem and progenitor cells.[90] In most of the reported models, a large segmental defect created in a long bone was filled with a cylinder of porous bioceramic carrying autologous, in-vitro-expanded, osteogenic progenitors. When stromal osteoprogenitors were locally delivered with the bioceramic scaffolds, stem cells efficiently promoted the healing of bone defects of critical sizes. Several clinical trials are underway to regenerate bone in humans after these successful results in animals.[91] New knowledge about stem and progenitor cells and their function in tissue regeneration provides a strong basis for using them to manage craniofacial defects.

Stem Cells in Cartilage Engineering

Artificial cartilage fabricated in vitro using tissue engineering has been applied to the repair and regeneration of damaged cartilage.[92] Various studies have shown that bone marrow-derived MSCs are more promising candidates for cartilage and bone tissue engineering than are primary chondrocytes or osteocytes, which are difficult to culture and expand.[93] Progenitor cells proliferate and differentiate into chondrocytes after implantation into the defect, which is important for regenerating enough cartilage to fill the defects. On the other hand, complete restoration of cartilage is not possible so far, and the newly formed cartilage within the surrounding host tissue is required to differentiate into fully matured chondrocytes. The combination of MSC-based cell therapy and gene transfer of selected differentiating cytokines may help in this challenge.[67]

Stem Cells in Wound Healing

Endothelial progenitor cell therapy and therapeutic vasculogenesis have various implications for plastic surgery. Recently, endothelial progenitor cell transplantation has been used to increase neovascularization in the problem areas.[94] After injection into the systemic circulation, endothelial progenitor cells reportedly selectively localized to the ischemic tissues; thus, these endothelial progenitor cells may be important in salvaging ischemic flaps. Therefore, therapeutic vasculogenesis has the potential to improve flap survival, improve wound healing, accelerate tissue expansion, and facilitate tissue engineering. Endothelial stem and progenitor cells may be useful for treating complicated wounds, such as those in patients with diabetes or from burns, replacing cells rather than growth factors alone.

Stem Cells in Tendon Engineering

In various experiments fibroblasts or bone marrow-derived mesenchymal stem cells were implanted into type I collagen gels to improve tendon and ligament repair.[95] Although biochemical and histological analyses revealed improved tissue architecture, more research is needed to improve the biomechanical properties and functionality of the injured tendon and to assure complete healing of the tendon and ligament defects. The use of exogenous growth factors may improve the success of tendon and ligament tissue engineering.

The Future of Stem Cells

Advances in gene-modifying techniques may allow stem cells to be modified during their ex vivo expansion; thus, it may be possible to make a patient's own stem cells even better. For example, in a genetic disease, replacing a missing gene activity or silencing a defective gene activity may become possible. Moreover, autologous stem and progenitor cells harvested from an individual and used for self-tissue repair is immunologically ideal. However, despite the great potential that stem and progenitor cells offer for treating many diseases and defects, many challenges remain:

1. *All stem cells have to be differentiated before transplantation can be successful*; otherwise, the presence of even a single undifferentiated stem cell that retains the capability to continuously reproduce may result in tumor formation.

2. When differentiated stem cells are not recognized as "self" by the recipient's immune system after an allogeneic transplantation, an immunologic response may prevent incorporation of the donor cells. In this case, stem cells could be individualized with genetic modifications, or immunosuppressive therapy could be used in conjunction with the transplanted cells. Having a large pool of stem and progenitor cells with different major histocompatibility complex backgrounds and using the most appropriate ones for the transplantation could be another solution.

3. Although some mesenchymal lineage-inducing agents are known, the molecular details regulating the lineage development need to be investigated. The genotype of each individual determines the secretion of growth factors and cytokines.[89] In addition, MSC cultures show donor-specific levels of cytokines. Thus, tissue engineering applications may necessitate patient-specific doses of lineage-stimulating and lineage-regulating factors.[89]

4. Some other problems in stem cell therapy include determining how, where, and when to introduce stem cell derivatives into a recipient; whether the potential of these cells will change over time; whether structural scaffolds are required to get the desired form; whether the imprinting status of cells derived from embryonic stem cells differs from adult cells; and how to efficiently differentiate or genetically tailor ESCs into the quantity needed for transplantation before the recipient's disease has progressed too far.[96]

References

1. Jacobson LO, Marks EK, Robson MJ, et al. Effect of spleen protection on mortality following x-irradiation. *J Lab Clin Med.* 1949;34:1538–1543.
2. Lorenz E, Uphoff D, Reid TR, et al. Modification of irradiation injury in mice and guinea pigs by bone marrow injections. *J Natl Cancer Inst.* 1951;12:197–201.
3. Till JE, McCulloch EA. A direct measurement of the radiation sensitivity of normal mouse bone marrow cells. *Radiat Res.* 1961;14:213–222.

4. Smith LG, Weissman IL, Heimfeld S. Clonal analysis of hematopoietic stem-cell differentiation in vivo. *Proc Natl Acad Sci USA*. 1991;88:2788–2792.

5. Uchida N, Weissman IL. Searching for hematopoietic stem cells: evidence that Thy-1.1 low Lin–Sca-1 cells are the only stem cells in C57BL/Ka-Thy-1.1 bone marrow. *J Exp Med*. 1992;175:175–184.

6. Andrews RG, Singer JW, Bernstein ID. Precursors of colony-forming cells in humans can be distinguished from colony-forming cells by expression of the CD33 and CD34 antigens and light scatter properties. *Blood*. 1986;67:842–858.

7. Baumhueter S, Dybdal N, Kyle C, et al. Global vascular expression of murine CD34, a sialomucin-like enodthelial ligand for L-selectin. *Blood*. 1994; 84:2554–2561.

8. Craig W, Kay R, Cutler RL, et al. Expression of Thy-1 on human hematopoietic progenitor cells. *J Exp Med*. 1993;177:1331–1342.

9. Thomas ED, Storb R. Technique for human marrow grafting. Blood 1970;36:507–515.

10. Areman EM, Deeg HJ, Sacher RA. *Bone Marrow and Stem Cell Processing: A Manual of Current Techniques*. Philadelphia: F.A. Davis & Co., 1992.

11. Kernan NA, Flomenberg N, Dupont B, et al. Graft rejection in recipients of T-cell-depleted HLA-nonidentical marrow transplants for leukemia. *Transplantation*. 1987;43:842–847.

12. Fliedner TM, Steinbach KH. Repopulating potential of hematopoietic precursor cells. *Blood Cells*. 1988;14:393–410.

13. Goldman JM, Th'ing KH, Park DS, et al. Collection, cryopreservation and subsequent viability of haemopoietic stem cells intended for treatment of chronic granulocytic leukemia in blast-cell transformation. *Br J Haematol*. 1978;40:185–188.

14. Valdimarsson H, Moss PD, Holt PJ, Hobbs JR. Treatment of chronic mucocutaneous candidiasis with leucocytes from HL-A compatible sibling. *Lancet*. 1972;1:469–472.

15. McNiece IK, Stewart FM, Deacon DM, et al. Detection of a human CFC with a high proliferative potential. *Blood*. 1989;74:609–612.

16. Demirer T, Buckner CD, Bensinger WI. Optimization of peripheral blood stem cell mobilization. *Stem Cells*. 1996;14(1):106–116.

17. Hohaus S, Goldschmidt H, Ehrhardt R, et al. Successful autografting following myeloablative conditioning therapy with blood stem cells mobilized by chemotherapy plus RHG-CSF. *Exp Hematol*. 1993;21:4: 508–514.

18. Dreger P, Marquardt P, Haferlach T, et al. Effective mobilization of peripheral blood progenitor cells with Dexa-BEAM and G-CSF-timing of harvesting and composition of the leukapheresis product. *Br J Cancer*. 1993;68:5:950–957.

19. Jagannath S, Vesole DH, Glenn L, Crowley J, Barlogie B. Low-risk intensive therapy for multiple myeloma with combined autologous bone marrow and blood stem cell support. *Blood*. 1992;80:1666–1672.

20. Shpall EJ, Jones RB, Bearman SI, et al. Transplantation of enriched CD34-positive autologous marrow into breast cancer patients following high-dose chemotherapy: influence of CD34-positive peripheral-blood progenitors and growth factors on engraftment. *J Clin Oncol*. 1994;12:28–36.

21. Kawano Y, Takaue Y, Watanabe T, Saito S, Abe T, Hirao A, et al. Effects of progenitor cell dose and preleukapheresis use of human recombinant granulocyte colony-stimulating factor on the recovery of hematopoiesis after blood stem cell autografting in children. *Exp Hematol*. 1993;21:103–108.

22. Storek J, Gooley T, Siadak M, Bensinger WI, Maloney DG, Chauncey TR, et al. Allogeneic peripheral blood stem cell transplantation may be associated with a high risk of chronic graft-versus-host disease. *Blood*. 1997; 90(12):4705–4709.

23. Bensinger WI, Weaver CH, Appelbaum FR, Rowley S, Demirer T, Sanders J, et al. Transplantation of allogeneic peripheral blood stem cells mobilized by recombinant human granulocyte colony-stimulating factor. *Blood*. 1995;85:1655–1658.

24. Schmitz N, Dreger P, Suttorp M, Rohwedder EB, Haferlach T, Loffler H, et al. Primary transplantation of allogeneic peripheral blood progenitor cells mobilized by filgrastim (granulocyte colony-stimulating factor). *Blood*. 1995;85:1666–1672.

25. Majolino I, Saglio G, Scime R, Serra A, Cavallaro AM, Fiandaca T, et al. High incidence of chronic GVHD after primary allogeneic peripheral blood stem cell transplantation in patients with hematologic malig-nancies. *Bone Marrow Transplant*. 1996;17:555–560.

26. Korbling M, Huh YO, Durett A, et al. Allogeneic blood stem cell transplantation: peripheralization and yield of donor-derived primitive hematopoietic progenitor cells (CD34+ Thy-1dim) and lymphoid subsets, and possible predictors of engraftment and GVHD. *Blood*. 1995; 86:2842–2848.

27. Indovina A, Majolino I, Scime R, et al. High dose cyclophosphamide: stem cell mobilizing capacity in 21 patients. *Leuk Lymphoma*. 1994;14:1–2:71–77.

28. Bensinger WI, Price TH, Dale DC, et al. The effects of daily recombinant human granulocyte colony-stimulating factor administration on normal granulocyte donors undergoing leukapheresis. *Blood*. 1993; 81:1883–1888.

29. Korbling M, Champlin R. Peripheral blood progenitor cell transplantation: a replacement for marrow auto- or allografts. *Stem Cells*. 1996;14:185–195.

30. Korbling M, Fliedner TM, Pflieger H. Collection of large quantities of granulocyte macrophage progenitor cells (CFUc) in man by means of continuous-flow leukapheresis. *Scand J Haematol*. 1980;24:22–28.

31. Chao NJ, Schriber JR, Grimes K, et al. Granulocyte colony-stimulating factor "mobilized" peripheral blood progenitor cells accelerate granulocyte and platelet recovery after high-dose chemotherapy. *Blood*. 1993; 81:2031–2035.

32. Ilhan O, Arslan Ö, Arat M, et al. The impact of the CD34+ cell dose on engraftment in allogeneic peripheral blood stem cell transplantation. *Transfus Sci*. 1999; 20:69–71.

33. Runde V, de Witte T, Arnold R, et al. Bone marrow transplantation from HLA-identical siblings as first-line treatment in patients with myelodysplastic syndromes: early transplantation is associated with improved outcome. *Bone Marrow Transp*. 1998;21:255–261.

34. Goldman JM. Modern approaches to the management of chronic granulocytic leukemia. *Semin Hematol*. 1978;15:420–430.

35. To LB, Haylock DN, Simmons PJ, Juttner CA. The biology and clinical uses of blood stem cells. *Blood.* 1997;89(7): 2233–2258.

36. Taichman RS, Emerson SG. The role of osteoblasts in the hematopoietic microenvironment. *Stem Cells.* 1998; 16(1):7–15.

37. Briscoe DM, Dharnidharka VR, Isaacs C, et al. The allogeneic response to cultured human skin equivalent in the hu-PBL-SCID mouse model of skin rejection. *Transplantation.* 1999;67:1590–1599.

38. Wiles MV, Keller G.Multiple hematopoietic lineages develop from embryonic stem (ES) cells in culture. *Development.* 1991;111(2):259–267.

39. Slager HG, Van Inzen W, Freund E, Van den Eijnden-Van Raaij AJ, Mummery CL. Transforming growth factor-beta in the early mouse embryo: implications for the regulation of muscle formation and implantation. *Dev Genet.* 1993;14(3):212–224.

40. Evans MJ, Kaufman MH. Establishment in culture of pluripotential cells from mouse embryos. *Nature.* 1981;292(5819):154–156.

41. Potocnik AJ, Kohler H, Eichmann K. Hemato-lymphoid in vivo reconstitution potential of subpopulations derived from in vitro differentiated embryonic stem cells. *Proc Natl Acad Sci USA.* 1997;94:10295–10300.

42. Lee SH, Lumelsky N, Studer L, et al. Efficient generation of midbrain and hindbrain neurons from mouse embryonic stem cells. *Nat Biotechnol.* 2000;18:675–679.

43. Klug MG, Soonpaa MH, Koh GY, et al. Genetically selected cardiomyocytes from differentiating embryonic stem cells form stable intracardiac grafts. *J Clin Invest.* 1996;98:216–224.

44. Ng WA, Doetschman T, Robbins J, et al. Muscle isoactin expression during in vitro differentiation of murine embryonic stem cells. *Pediatr Res.* 1997;41:285–292.

45. Strom TB, Field LJ, Ruediger M. Allogeneic stem Cells, clinical transplantation, and the origins of regenerative medicine. *Curr Opin Immunol.* 2002;14(5):601–605.

46. Gluckman E, Rocha V, Boyer-Chammard A, et al. Outcome of cord-blood transplantation from related and unrelated donors. *N Engl J Med.* 1997;337:373–281.

47. McCullough J, Herr G, Lennon S, et al. Factors influencing the availability of umbilical cord blood for banking and transplantation. *Transfusion.* 1998;38:508–510.

48. Donaldson C, Armitage WJ, Buchanan RM, et al. Obstetric factors influencing cord blood collections. *Blood.* 1998;92:121a.

49. Shlebak AA, Roberts IAG, Stevens TA, et al. The impact of antenatal and perinatal variables on cord blood haemopoietic stem/progenitor cell yield available for transplantation. *Br J Haematol.* 1998;103:1167–1171.

50. McCullough J, Herr G, Lennon S, et al. Factors influencing the availability of umbilical cord blood for banking and transplantation. *Transfusion.* 1998;38:508–510.

51. Broxmeyer HE, Douglas GW, Hangoc G, et al. Human umbilical cord blood as a potential source of transplantable hematopoietic stem/progenitor cells. *Proc Natl Acad Sci USA.* 1989;86:3828–3832.

52. Gluckman E, Broxmeyer HE, Auerbach AD, et al. Hematopoietic reconstitution in a patient with Fanconi's anemia by means of umbilical-cord blood from an HLA-identical sibling. *N Engl J Med.* 1989;321:1174–1178.

53. Miller AD, Buttimore C. Redesign of retrovirus packaging cell lines to avoid recombination leading to helper virus production. *Mol Cell Biol.* 1986;6:2895–2902.

54. Dunbar CE, Emmons RV. Gene transfer into hematopoietic progenitor and stem cells: progress and problems. *Stem Cells.* 1994;12:563–576.

55. Williams DA. Ex vivo expansion of hematopoietic stem and progenitor cells—robbing Peter to pay Paul. *Blood.* 1993;81:3169–3172.

56. Bhatia M, Bonnet D, Kapp U, et al. Quantitative analysis reveals expansion of human hematopoietic repopulating cells after short-term ex vivo culture. *J Exp Med.* 1997;186:619–624.

57. Shimakura Y, Kawada H, Ando K, Sato T, Nakamura Y, Tsuji T, et al. Murine stromal cell line HESS-5 maintains reconstituting ability of ex vivo-generated hematopoietic stem cells from human bone marrow and cytokine-mobilized peripheral Blood. *Stem Cells.* 2000;18(3): 183–189.

58. Hanazono Y, Terao K, Ozawa K. Gene transfer into non-human primate hematopoietic stem cells: implications for gene therapy. *Stem Cells.* 2001;19(1):12–23.

59. Kurre P, Kiem HP, Morris J, et al. Efficient transduction by an amphotropic retrovirus vector is dependent on the high-level expression of the cell surface virus receptor. *J Virol.* 1999;73:495–500.

60. Brossart P, Wirths S, Brugger W, Kanz L. Dendritic cells in cancer vaccines. *Exp Hematol.* 2001;29: 1247–1255.

61. Orlic D, Kajstura J, Chimenti S, et al. Bone marrow cells regenerate infarcted mouse myocardium. *Nature.* 2001; 410:701–705.

62. Ferrari G, Cusella-De Angelis G, Coletta M, et al. Muscle regeneration by bone marrow derived myogenic progenitors. *Science.* 1998;279:1528–1530.

63. Mezey E, Chandross K, Harta G, et al. Turning blood in brain: cells bearing neuronal antigens generated in vivo from bone marrow. *Science.* 2000;290:1779–1782.

64. Lagasse E, Connors H, Al-Dhalimy M, et al. Purified hematopoietic stem cells can differentiate into hepatocytes in vivo. *Nature Med.* 2000;6:1229–1234.

65. Krause D, Theise N, Collector M, et al. Multi-organ, multi-lineage engraftment by a single bone marrow-derived stem cell. *Cell.* 2001;105:369–377.

66. Jackson KA, Majka SM, Wang H, et al. Regeneration of ischemic cardiac muscle and vascular endothelium by adult stem cells. *J Clin Invest.* 2001;107:1395–1402.

67. Ringe J, Kaps C, Burmester GR, Sittinger M.. Stem cells for regenerative medicine: advances in the engineering of tissues and organs.*Naturwissenschaften.* 2002;89:338–51.

68. Vogel G. Can adult stem cells suffice? *Science.* 2001; 292:1820–1822.

69. Bianco P, Riminucci M, Gronthos S, et al. Bone marrow stromal stem cells: nature, biology, and potential applications. *Stem Cells.* 2001;19:180–192.

70. Colter DC, Class R, DiGirolamo CM, et al. Rapid expansion of recycling stem cells in cultures of plastic-adherent cells from human bone marrow. *Proc Natl Acad Sci USA.* 2000;97:3213–3218.

71. Campagnoli C, Roberts IAG, Kumar S, et al. Identification of mesenchymal stem/progenitor cells in human first-trimester fetal blood, liver, and bone marrow. *Blood.* 2001;98:2396–2402.

72. Tilney NL, Whitley WD, Diamond JR. Chronic rejection: an unidentified conundrum. *Transplantation.* 1991; 52:389–398.

73. Dunn DL. Problems related to immunosuppression. Infection and malignancy occurring after solid organ transplantation. *Crit Care Clin.* 1990;6:955–957.

74. Pittenger MF, Mackay AM, Beck SC, Jaiswal RK, Douglas R, Mosca JD, et al. Multilineage potential of adult human mesenchymal stem cells. *Science.* 1999;284:143–147.

75. Rao MS, Mattson MP. Stem cells and aging: expanding the possibilities. *Mech Ageing Dev.* 2001;122:713–734.

76. Lee WP, Yaremchuk MJ, Pan YC, Randolph MA, Tan CM, Weiland AJ. Relative antigenicity of components of a vascularized limb allograft. *Plast Reconstr Surg.* 1991;87(3):401–411.

77. Benham P, Anthony JP, Ferreira L, Borsanyi JP, Mathes SJ. Use of combination of low-dose cyclosporine and RS-61443 in a rat hind limb model of composite tissue allotransplantation. *Transplantation.* 1996;61(4):527–532.

78. Foster RD, Ascher NL, McCalmont TH, Neipp M, Anthony JP, Mathes SJ. Mixed allogeneic chimerism as a reliable model for composite tissue allograft tolerance induction across major and minor histocompatibility barriers. *Transplantation.* 2001;72(5):791–797.

79. Sachs DH. Mixed chimerism as an approach to transplantation tolerance. *Clin Immunol.* 2000;95(1 Pt 2):63–68.

80. Fuchimoto Y, Yamada K, Shimizu A, Yasumoto A, Sawada T, Huang CH, et al. Relationship between chimerism and tolerance in a kidney transplantation model. *J Immunol.* 1999;162(10):5704–5711.

81. Siemionow M, Zielinski M, Ozmen S, Izycki D, Ozer K. Intraosseus injection of the donor-derived bone marrow stem and progenitor cells increase donor-specific chimerism and extends composite tissue allograft survival. *Transplant Proc.* In press.

82. Siemionow MZ, Izycki DM, Zielinski M. Donor-specific tolerance in fully major histocompatibility major histocompatibility complex-mismatched limb allograft transplants under an anti-alphabeta T-cell receptor monoclonal antibody and cyclosporine A protocol. *Transplantation.* 2003;76(12):1662–1668.

83. Takagi K, Urist MR. The role of bone marrow in bone morphogenetic protein-induced repair of femoral massive diaphyseal defects. *Clin Orthop Relat Res.* 1982;(171):224–231.

84. Carsin H, Ainaud P, Le Bever H, Rives J, Lakhel A, Stephanazzi J, et al. Cultured epithelial autografts in extensive burn coverage of severely traumatized patients: a five year single-center experience with 30 patients. *Burns.* 2000;26:379–387.

85. Peterson L, Minas T, Brittberg M, Lindahl A. Treatment of osteochondritis dissecans of the knee with autologous chondrocyte transplantation: results at two to ten years. *J Bone Joint Surg Am.* 2003;85-A suppl 2:17–24.

86. Tran N, Li Y, Bertrand S, Bangratz S, Carteaux JP, Stoltz JF, et al. Autologous cell transplantation and cardiac tissue engineering: potential applications in heart failure. *Biorheology.* 2003;40:411–415.

87. Binder S, Stolba U, Krebs I, Kellner L, Jahn C, Feichtinger H, et al. Transplantation of autologous retinal pigment epithelium in eyes with foveal neovascularization resulting from age-related macular degeneration: a pilot study. *Am J Ophthalmol.* 2002;133:215–225.

88. Cheng B, Chen Z. Fabricating autologous tissue to engineer artificial nerve. *Microsurgery.* 2002;22:133–137.

89. Caplan AI, Bruder SP. Mesenchymal stem cells: building blocks for molecular medicine in the 21st century. *Trends Mol Med.* 2001;7:259–264.

90. Kon E, Muraglia A, Corsi A, et al. Autologous bone marrow stromal cells loaded onto porous hydroxyapatite ceramic accelerate bone repair in critical-size defects of sheep long bones. *J Biomed Mater Res.* 2000;49:328–337.

91. Grzesik WJ, Cheng H, Oh JS, Kuznetsov SA, Mankani MH, Uzawa K, et al. Cementum-forming cells are phenotypically distinct from bone-forming cells. *J Bone Miner Res.* 2000;15(1):52–59.

92. Wakitani S, Goto T, Pineda SJ, et al. Mesenchymal cell-based repair of large, full-thickness defects of articular cartilage. *J Bone Joint Surg Am.* 1994;76:579–592.

93. Lee HS, Huang GT, Chiang H, Chiou LL, Chen MH, Hsieh CH, et al. Multipotential mesenchymal stem cells from femoral bone marrow near the site of osteonecrosis. *Stem Cells.* 2003;21:190–199.

94. Cairo MS, Wagner JE. Placental and/or umbilical cord blood: an alternative source of hematopoietic stem cells for transplantation. *Blood.* 1997;90:4665–4678

95. Awad HA, Butler DL, Harris MT, Ibrahim RE, Wu Y, Young RG, et al. In vitro characterization of mesenchymal stem cell-seeded collagen scaffolds for tendon repair: effects of initial seeding density on contraction kinetics. *J Biomed Mater Res.* 2000;51:233–240.

96. Pfendler KC, Kawase E. The potential of stem cells. *Obstet Gynecol Sur.* 2003;58(3):197–208.

Index